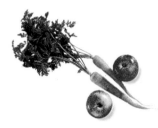

Health And Healing
The Natural Way

Eating for Good Health

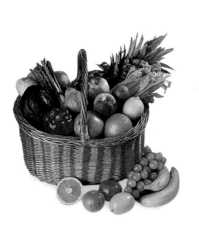

HEALTH AND HEALING
THE NATURAL WAY

EATING FOR GOOD HEALTH

PUBLISHED BY

THE READER'S DIGEST ASSOCIATION LIMITED

LONDON NEW YORK SYDNEY MONTREAL CAPE TOWN

EATING FOR GOOD HEALTH
was created and produced by
Carroll & Brown Limited
20 Lonsdale Road, London NW6 6RD
for The Reader's Digest Association Limited, London

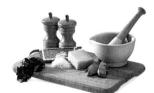

CARROLL & BROWN

Managing Editor Denis Kennedy
Art Director Chrissie Lloyd

Series Editor Arlene Sobel
Series Art Editor Johnny Pau

Editor Patricia Shine
Assistant Editor Melanie Halton

Art Editor Mercedes Morgan
Designer Michelle Tiley

Photographers David Murray, Jules Selmes

Production Lorraine Baird, Wendy Rogers,
Amanda Mackie

Computer Management John Clifford, Caroline Turner

First English Edition Copyright © 1995
The Reader's Digest Association Limited,
11 Westferry Circus, Canary Wharf,
London E14 4HE

Reprinted with amendments 1999

Copyright © 1995
Reader's Digest Association Far East Limited
Philippines Copyright © 1995
Reader's Digest Association Far East Limited

ISBN 0 276 42194 9

Reproduced by Colourscan, Singapore
Printing and binding: Printer Industria Gráfica S.A., Barcelona

CONSULTANTS

Professor Tom Sanders BSc, PhD
Department of Nutrition & Dietetics
School of Life, Basic Medical & Health Sciences
King's College, University of London

Dr Paul Lachance
Department of Food Science, Cook College
Rutgers University, New Brunswick, New Jersey, USA

Moya de Wet BSc, SRD
Consultant Nutritionist
State Registered Dietitian

MEDICAL ILLUSTRATIONS CONSULTANT

Dr Frances Williams MB, BChir,
MRCP, DTM&H

CONTRIBUTORS

Anita Bean BSC

Roger Newman-Turner BAc, ND, DO, MRO, MRN
Registered naturopath, osteopath and acupuncturist

Lyndel Costain BSc
State Registered Dietitian

Dr Lesley Hickin MB, BS, BSc,
DRCOG, MRCGP

FOR READER'S DIGEST

Series Editor Christine Noble
Editorial Assistant Caroline Boucher

READER'S DIGEST GENERAL BOOKS

Editorial Director Cortina Butler
Art Director Nick Clark

The information in this book is for reference only;
it is not intended as a substitute for a doctor's diagnosis and care.
The editors urge anyone with continuing medical problems
or symptoms to consult a doctor.

EATING FOR GOOD HEALTH

More and more people today are choosing to take greater responsibility for their own health rather than relying on the doctor to step in with a cure when something goes wrong. We now recognise that we can influence our health by making an improvement in lifestyle – a better diet, more exercise and reduced stress. People are also becoming increasingly aware that there are other healing methods – some new, others very ancient – that can help to prevent illness or be used as a complement to orthodox medicine.
The series *Health and Healing the Natural Way* will help you to make your own health choices by giving you clear, comprehensive, straightforward and encouraging information and advice about methods of improving your health. The series explains the many different natural therapies now available – aromatherapy, herbalism, acupressure and many others – and the many circumstances in which they may be of benefit when used in conjunction with conventional medicine.

In *EATING FOR GOOD HEALTH* you will find out just how much your health and general well-being is determined by what you eat and how even a minor change in your diet can help to strengthen your resistance to many illnesses from the common cold to heart disease, cancer, hypertension and stroke. You will find out how to assess every aspect of your present diet and understand the different part played in a healthy diet by protein, carbohydrates, fibre, fats and minerals. The book highlights aspects of the diets of different countries that may be usefully incorporated into a healthy diet. And there are practical suggestions to help you make the changes in your diet and that of every family member that will enable you to reap the ultimate benefit – a long and healthy life.

CONTENTS

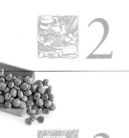
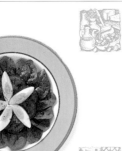

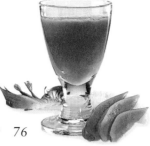

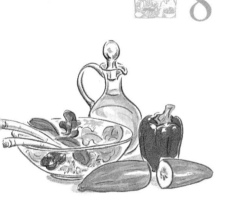

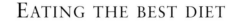

FOOD AND HEALTH – THE VITAL LINK

The alliance of modern chemistry with statistical surveys is leading to a new understanding of how what we eat affects both short and long-term health.

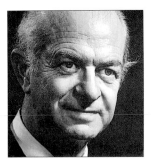

LINUS PAULING
The American chemist, Dr Linus Pauling (1901–94), put forward the idea in 1970 of using vitamin C to cure the common cold. Since then, many studies have tested its validity but with little success. Yet research shows that vitamin C helps the body to fight infection.

DISCOVERY OF VITAMINS
For centuries people suffered debilitating diseases, such as scurvy and beriberi, which are caused by vitamin deficiencies. When the first vitamin was recognised for its special properties in 1912, it was named A, and subsequent finds were named after the following letters of the alphabet.

It seems almost absurd to state that you need food to live. The body has a very potent built-in alarm signal – hunger – to tell you when your supply of food, the 'fuel for the body', is low and thereby ensure that you are never in serious danger of forgetting to eat. One of the most fascinating aspects of the way the body works is that this alarm signal is also choosy and at times asks for specific supplies, for example, sweet things when your body sugar is low or water when you are thirsty.

What many people fail to recognise is that their bodies have more than just one signal. Tiredness, looking and feeling run down, aches and pains, stress, even chronic disease – all these can be indications of a diet that is lacking nutrition. But not all of these signals are instant or 'colour-coded' for easy reference, and that is the heart of the problem. Since no one can see or experience the results of a bad diet immediately (often the effects take years to develop), few people realise just how closely bodily health is linked to what they eat, how much they eat and how often they eat. You are what you eat, and the food you eat affects the way you feel and the way you look all through your life.

A 20TH-CENTURY CONUNDRUM

Science over the past 100 years has made immense strides in medical knowledge and the treatment of illness, with the result that average life spans have gradually extended since the turn of the century. However, at the same time that a number of infectious diseases have been eradicated, and when technological advances in sanitation, immunisation, surgery and genetic engineering are increasing life expectancies, the incidence of chronic disorders like cancer and heart disease has quietly shot up. It is even more incongruous that the main victims of these modern plagues live in the Western industrialised countries, the very areas where medical research is most advanced.

Medical scientists are now quite certain that diet is at the root of most heart disease. The human body is not equipped to cope with the modern diet, which is often too high in fat and too low in complex carbohydrates. Because insufficient food has been, until modern times, mankind's greatest concern, the body has developed to extract the maximum out of the minimum, making the best use of available seasonal supplies. The body lays down fat in periods of plenty in order to survive during lean times. But today the main problem for most people in developed countries is excess rather than dearth, and the effects of this imbalance are proving to be equally dangerous. If diet is the cause of illness, however, it is fortunately also the cure.

THE NEW SCIENTIFIC CONSENSUS

Just a few years ago, the idea that heart disease, osteoporosis and cancer could be treated in the kitchen was considered quackery. The discovery of wonder drugs and antibiotics after the Second World War brought a change in the way medicine was practised and the body was perceived. As the achievements of laboratory medicine became ever more complex, treatment became concentrated in the hands of specialists who focused on specific aspects of the body. The real medicines were seen as being pills and potions, not herbs and other natural remedies. Nature, in the form of the raw material of life – food – could not compete with the specialist's skills.

But once scientists discovered that the high-fibre, low-fat diet eaten in non-industrialised countries seemed to give protection against certain chronic illnesses, the preventive powers of food and diet slowly came to be recognised once more. Certainly, changes in diets can save lives. Since the 1970s deaths in the United Kingdom from coronary artery disease have fallen by more than 20 per cent, in part because people are eating less fat and cholesterol. But many people still do not know what food can do for them after it has suppressed hunger pangs. Old wives' tales about carrots helping you

A VEGETARIAN DIET
Many famous characters throughout history have advocated a vegetarian diet – the Florentine painter Leonardo da Vinci (1452–1519), the American statesman and scientist Benjamin Franklin (1706–90), the Irish dramatist George Bernard Shaw (1856–1950) and the Indian political leader Mahatma Gandhi (1869–1948) all abstained from eating meat. The reasons for becoming vegetarian may be religious, ethical, health-related or environmental.

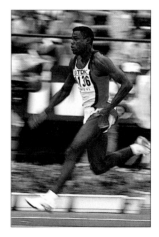

CARL LEWIS
The American track and field athlete, Carl Lewis (b. 1961), follows a strict vegetarian diet. Lewis won four gold medals in the 1984 Olympics.

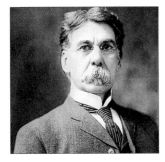

to see in the dark, spinach building up your muscles or fish sharpening your brains have proved not far wrong and triggered research leading to greater scientific knowledge about the properties of food and the way your body uses it. Each of the 100 trillion cells in your body undergoes billions of chemical reactions every second, and your health may depend on whether a particular enzyme, vitamin or mineral is able to come to the rescue at the right moment. The foods you eat possess powerful capabilities to help and to harm.

ARE YOU KEEPING IN TOUCH WITH THE NEW FOOD FACTS?

Research into the health implications of food is advancing at a furious pace. Some findings are by now well known – that you should eat fresh foods and cut down on fat, for example. But do you know the latest findings that may be crucial to your health and the health of your family? For instance, do you know that eating oily fish helps to thin the blood and prevent clots? That garlic may have special anti-cancer properties? And what about the 'Food Pyramid'? Do you understand the recommendations for healthy eating?

The power of food to swing the balance of health one way or another is remarkable. Substances in some foods are toxic, such as the solanine found in sprouting potatoes. Other substances fight toxins, such as certain compounds found in cabbage that may help to combat the detrimental effects of cancer-causing pollutants in the body. The influence of food on heart disease is particularly well documented. Some types of food may cause the build up of plaque in the arteries, causing them to clog; other foods release substances that scrub the arteries clean. Saturated fat, for example, is the source for the synthesis of artery-clogging cholesterol in the liver, while soluble fibre, such as is found in oat bran or beans, has been shown to bind intestinal cholesterol, thus helping the body to excrete it.

Foods can both promote cancer development and help to prevent it. Raw mushrooms, for example, contain hydrazines, and peanuts can carry aflatoxin from mould contamination – both of which are known carcinogens. Eaten regularly over a lifetime, substances in spinach, broccoli and cauliflower have been linked to cancer prevention, as has an acid found in certain types of berries.

It is therefore not surprising that some medical conditions are treated through dietary changes. The treatment of gout includes instructions to eat less offal and drink less alcohol, and management of diabetes mellitus demands control of the carbohydrates consumed. There is hardly a bodily process or disorder that is untouched in some way by what you put in your mouth.

INCREASING YOUR UNDERSTANDING OF FOOD

Every day seems to bring an avalanche of statistics and new diets to match them. A recent survey of English-language women's magazines showed that on average a new healthy or slimming diet was published in every third issue, only to be cancelled out three issues later by one claiming to be more effective. Various foods can become the panacea or poison of the month. One dietary fad may subject the body to total abstention from selected foods, another may demand that certain foods should be eaten in unusual quantities. At times, food is granted second place altogether to vitamin pills and other nutritional supplements, in the belief that these may provide short cuts to good nutrition.

But a miracle or fad diet is not the solution, nor are megadoses of vitamin pills. Scientists now know that food and its effects are every bit as complex as our own bodies. Of the thousands of chemicals, minerals and vitamins found in a single food, many are potential life-savers or hazards to health, depending on how much is consumed over time. Here the old adage of variety being the spice of life is proving wiser than anyone ever knew. Eating a variety of foods means that you are more likely to get a good supply of adequate nutrients, since anything lacking in one food will be supplied in another. The link between food and health is an everyday but complex issue. So, rather than trusting in fads, you should learn how to balance your food intake. Small but well-informed changes to your diet will make a great difference to your well-being.

EATING YOUR WAY TO GOOD HEALTH

The aim of EATING FOR GOOD HEALTH is to help you do just that – to think about the food you eat and ask yourself whether you are doing the sensible thing for yourself and your family. On the sound principle that self-education is superior to following fashionable trends when making sound food choices, EATING FOR GOOD HEALTH leads you through the many layers of contemporary living where food occupies a key role – inside the body and in the kitchen, the laboratory, the factory and the market place.

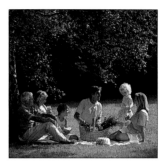

GENERATIONS OF
HEALTHY EATERS
The kinds of food you eat and how often you eat them, have a major influence on your emotional and physical development. Much of the way people eat depends on habits fixed since childhood, but it is never too late to start eating a healthy diet. Whatever your age, you will always need a good supply of nutrients, and this is easily found in a well-balanced, varied diet.

'TO YOUR HEALTH'
Drinking fresh fruit juice will help you to increase your intake of vitamin C. One 175 ml (6 fl oz) glass of orange juice meets your daily need of vitamin C.

Chapter 1 will help you to understand why good eating habits can keep you healthy. You will learn how often and how much to eat, and how to identify the signs of nutritional imbalance.

Chapters 2 to 5 explore how your body uses the essential nutrients: proteins, carbohydrates, fats, vitamins and minerals. You will learn how much of these nutrients the foods you eat contain, and how to regulate and balance your nutritional intake. Chapter 2 also highlights the importance for vegetarians of combining plant foods to achieve a good intake of protein.

The body is even more sensitive to an imbalance in fluid than one in solid food. Chapter 6 details the body's requirements and evaluates the types of fluid you drink.

HEALTHY EATING FROM FARM TO TABLE

The past 40 years have seen a revolution for consumers, with the rise on the one hand of increased use of chemicals for pest control, fertilising and preservation and on the other hand of chemical-free organic farming. But increased choice in packaging, processing and farming techniques is in itself no guarantee of a good diet. It is important, therefore, to be able to distinguish healthful foods from junk foods and foods that may be harmful. Chapter 7 provides detailed information to help you make the best choices.

Chapter 8 evaluates diets from countries around the world and shows you how to take advantage of the Mediterranean, Japanese and Chinese styles of eating. This chapter also explores the requirements of people with special dietary needs including toddlers, pregnant women, diabetes sufferers and people with high blood pressure. By matching your diet to your lifestyle and developing better eating habits both at home and when you eat out, you can keep yourself in the best of health.

Chapter 9 tells you how to prepare foods for maximum nutritional value and stock up on the basics for a healthy diet. This chapter also outlines up-to-date information on long-term storage and preservation, refrigeration and thawing, and the optimum cooking methods for freshness, nutritional value and safety from the dangers of food poisoning.

EATING FOR GOOD HEALTH is designed to help you and your family understand more about the nature of the food you eat and the essential role of nutrition in the wider context of health, the promotion of physical and emotional well-being and the proper balancing of the social pleasures of the table with the vital requirements of the body.

ARE YOU EATING FOR GOOD HEALTH?

You may feel reasonably healthy and think that you are eating the right things but, nationally, statistics are saying otherwise. On a daily basis, the average UK citizen eats just over half the amount of fruit recommended by the World Health Organization and almost double the recommended intake of fat.

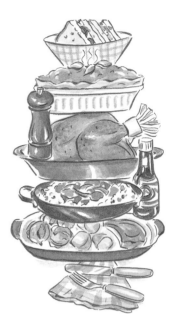

Q HOW MANY MEALS DO YOU EAT DURING THE DAY?

Do you usually eat one meal, two to three meals, or three or more meals a day? Eating one large feast a day is not very healthy. Nor is it any better to have a varying number of mealtimes from day to day. Your body works much better with a regular supply of nutrients provided in three or four regularly spaced meals a day. In particular, avoid skipping breakfast because you will expose yourself all the more to the temptation of sugary or fatty snacks, which you may crave by mid morning. Chapter 1 gives you some pointers on how to schedule your mealtimes.

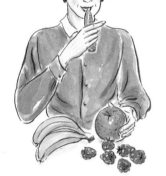

Q DO YOU EAT SNACKS BETWEEN MEALS?

Do you always snack between meals, now and again, or never?

In general, snacking is not a good habit to fall into if the snacks consist of sweets, savoury titbits and pastries that are high in calories and fats. If you know that you do succumb frequently to the urge, make sure that your snacks will add something to your diet rather than undoing it. For more tips on healthy ways to snack see Chapter 8.

Q HOW MANY SERVINGS OF FRUIT AND VEGETABLES DO YOU EAT EACH DAY?

Do you have one, two, or the recommended five servings a day? The fibre in fruit and vegetables comes as an important extra to their food value. Provided your intake of essential proteins and fats is met, you would be hard put to eat too much fruit or too many vegetables. Some of the more impressive benefits of fruits and vegetables are listed in Chapters 5 and 7.

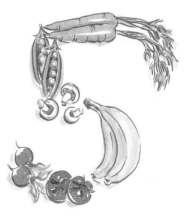

Q HOW OFTEN DO YOU EAT CARBOHYDRATE FOODS WITH YOUR MEALS?

Is it less, or more, than once a day? Complex-carbohydrate foods, such as bread, rice, potatoes, cereals and pasta – particularly if unrefined –

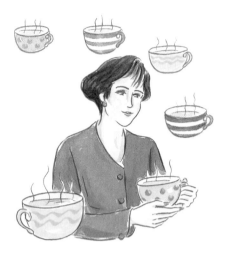

should make up at least half of your daily calorie intake. You should avoid adding high-calorie sauces to pasta and potatoes. The role of carbohydrates and ways of increasing the levels of fibre in your diet are discussed in Chapter 3.

Q HOW MANY CAFFEINATED DRINKS DO YOU TAKE PER DAY?

Do you have fewer than two drinks, from two to five drinks a day, or more? The benefit of caffeine is that it makes you alert, but this should be balanced by a moderation in its use, since it can raise blood pressure. Ideally, drink as little coffee and cola as possible and get out of the habit of using these drinks as an all-purpose liquid source. The advantages and disadvantages of caffeine are examined in Chapter 6.

Q HOW OFTEN DO YOU EAT RED MEATS?

Do you consume red meat twice a week, more than twice a week or every day? Red meats are high in saturated fat but they are also nutritionally important so, rather than eliminating them entirely, you should restrict your consumption to two meals with red meat a week. The value of meat and other rich sources of protein is illustrated in Chapter 2, and Chapter 4 details the types of fat that meats contain.

KEEPING A FOOD DIARY

Recording your daily food and drink intake is a very good way to monitor your present eating habits and to find out exactly what you eat. You may be asked to keep a food diary by a nutritionist, naturopath, dietitian, personal trainer, doctor or other health professional. This will enable them to gain a more accurate picture of your eating habits, compare your intake with the recommended values for protein, carbohydrate, fat, vitamins and minerals and advise you on any changes you need to make.

When filling in your food diary, describe the food as accurately as possible; for example, a cheese sandwich is actually three foods – bread, butter and cheese. Give a clear description of the type of food, such as whether the bread is wholemeal or white; the milk is skimmed, semi-skimmed, or full-fat; the spread is butter, margarine, low-fat spread, or mayonnaise. Include every spoonful of sugar in your coffee and every scrape of butter on your bread.

FILLING IN YOUR FOOD DIARY
Write down everything you eat and drink for at least three consecutive days. Make sure that you include one weekend day. Take the diary with you if you eat away from home, for example in the office canteen.

Kitchen   **Alone**
7:30 a.m.
1 glass of orange juice
2 slices of white toast with butter

Office   **Friends**
11:00 a.m.
1 large cup of black coffee
1 large jam doughnut

Café   **Friends**
1:00 p.m.
6 pieces French bread with butter
85 g (3 oz) Cheddar cheese
2 tbsp coleslaw & 1 bottle of beer

Kitchen   **Alone**
7:30 p.m.
2 small lamb chops
115 g (4 oz) baked potato & 1 tsp butter
2 tbsp peas
1 glass of white wine

Lounge   **Husband**
9:30 p.m.
1 cup of coffee with semi-skimmed milk, and 1 chocolate bar

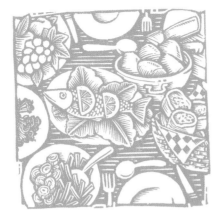

CHAPTER 1

HEALTHY EATING

*Not too many years ago, the optimum
diet was said to be one high in quality protein,
the kind found in animal foods. Today the advice is
to cut down on red meat because of its high content
of saturated fat. Moreover, experts advise, foods high
in complex carbohydrates and fibre – wholewheat
pasta, wholegrain bread, and brown rice – should,
along with plenty of fresh fruit and vegetables,
form the largest part of a healthy diet.*

ARE YOU EATING THE RIGHT FOODS?

Most people know that a well-balanced diet is vital for good health. Understanding your body's requirements and the foods that will meet them will enable you to make the right choices.

Think of your body as a mechanism made up of billions of tiny chemical factories linked in an endless process of utilising energy and performing such functions as nerve transmission and producing vital enzymes (body substances made from proteins that break down foods and regulate metabolism). Something as complicated as the human body must inevitably require differing varieties and amounts of resources to function. Fortunately, everything the average healthy person needs can be provided by a diet containing the right amount of proteins, carbohydrates, fats, fibre, minerals and vitamins. Each is essential to your well-being.

THE BODY'S NEEDS

Proteins are the key building materials in all cells and are needed for growth and cell replacement or repair. Eating meat, fish, eggs, grains, beans and dairy products will provide an ample supply of protein.

Carbohydrates are the body's fuel. They give you the energy to run a marathon as well as sustaining you during sleep. Even at rest, the body needs energy for growth, repairs and maintenance. Carbohydrates can be eaten in a variety of forms, from table sugar to bread, but for good health, foods containing complex carbohydrates – wholewheat pasta, for example – are best.

The carbohydrates in simple or refined sugars, like table sugar, or those found in chocolate bars, pastries, biscuits and cakes are absorbed quickly into the bloodsteam and are either used up rapidly or stored as fat in your body. Complex carbohydrates or starches, however, take time to break down into the simpler sugar units that your body's cells burn for energy. A slower, more steady flow of energy is released into your bloodstream ready to meet your needs.

Fats help to form the delicate membranes around and inside the body cells and act as carriers for the four fat-soluble vitamins A,

CHECKING LABELS
When choosing packaged products, read the labels carefully. Pay special attention to how much fat, sugar and sodium (salt) the food contains.

READING FOOD LABELS

Over the past 40 years, the range of foods available in packets, jars and cans has increased dramatically. Legislative bodies recognised that consumers required more information in order to make the best choices for health, which resulted in improved product labels.

Food manufacturers in the European Community and North America are required by law to provide the following information on product labels: total weight or volume, a list of the ingredients and of the additives in order of weight, the name and address of the manufacturer and the country of origin.

Manufacturers should also list caloric value per 100g, suggested number of servings the packaged food provides and the date after which the product cannot be sold or should not be eaten. This date is usually stamped on the lid or the base of products. Many labels also provide a nutritional analysis of food, such as total fat, carbohydrate and protein content.

D, E, K and other nutrients. Stored fat can be broken down and converted into sugars to provide the body with additional fuel.

Fibre, or roughage, is the indigestible part of foods. It is important because, in combination with the water you drink and the complex carbohydrates you eat, it provides the bulk needed to carry waste products speedily from your body. Low-fibre diets are associated with constipation, haemorrhoids and other more serious bowel problems, including colitis and possibly colon cancer. Good sources of fibre are cereals, grains, bran, fruits and vegetables.

The trillions of cells in your body need tiny amounts of minerals, such as copper, zinc, sodium, calcium and potassium to carry out their essential biochemical activities. A diet containing a variety of foods is the best way to obtain a good mix of these minerals. Your body also requires other special food substances called vitamins. These are needed only in relatively small amounts, but are essential for various vital functions. Vitamins release energy from food, help to make blood cells and hormones and maintain healthy organs and optimum functions of systems such as the nervous system.

Finally, water is vital for life – as the principal component of body fluids it carries nutrients around the body, lubricates joints and dissolves food for digestion and absorption. Water is contained in all the foods you eat, and the tea, coffee, milk and fruit juice you drink, but you should also drink plenty of plain water each day.

How food is digested

The nutrients your body needs for energy, maintenance and repair – including amino acids, glucose, fatty acids, vitamins and minerals – must first be extracted from food by the process of digestion.

Digestion begins in your mouth as you chew the food you are eating to break it up into smaller pieces. Chewing also stimulates the production of saliva, which contains enzymes that begin to break the food down chemically. Food combined with saliva passes through a long tube (pharynx and oesophagus) that stretches down your throat and chest and into the stomach. From there, the food goes through the small intestine (duodenum, jejunum and ileum) and the large intestine (caecum, colon and rectum). The tube ends at the anus.

MAKING THE RIGHT CHOICES

Different foods can provide similar nutrients. Most foods fall into one of four groupings, each of which provides a higher concentration of certain nutrients.

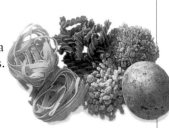

Meat, poultry, fish, nuts, eggs and pulses (beans, peas and lentils) are excellent sources of protein and also contain significant amounts of minerals and B vitamins

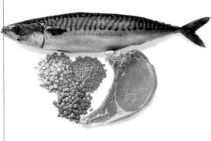

Wholemeal cereals, breads and pasta, brown rice and potatoes are rich in complex carbohydrates, contain some protein and are usually low in fats

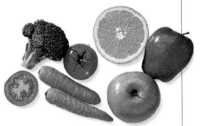

Dairy foods such as milk and low-fat cheese are excellent sources of quality protein, calcium, potassium and B vitamins. Full-fat varieties or fortified dairy products contain vitamins A and D

Fruits and vegetables are the best sources of fibre, minerals and vitamins. Have a variety daily as different fruits and vegetables contain varying combinations of vitamins and minerals

THE DIGESTIVE SYSTEM

As food travels through the system, it is broken down in various ways until all its nutritional value is absorbed. The remaining waste products are then expelled by the body.

Mouth – enzymes in saliva begin to break down starch

Pharynx and oesophagus – food passes through the tube to stomach

Stomach – gastric juices break down proteins

Small intestine – fats and carbohydrates and other nutrients are absorbed and passed to the bloodstream

Large intestine – water and salt are absorbed and waste matter is passed to the rectum

THE FOOD PYRAMID

In 1990, American government nutritionists developed the food pyramid to demonstrate how much food from the different groups needs to be eaten every day for a nutritionally balanced diet.

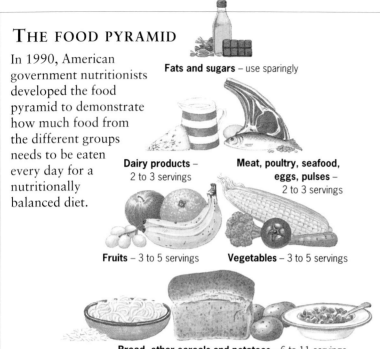

Fats and sugars – use sparingly

Dairy products – 2 to 3 servings

Meat, poultry, seafood, eggs, pulses – 2 to 3 servings

Fruits – 3 to 5 servings

Vegetables – 3 to 5 servings

Bread, other cereals and potatoes – 6 to 11 servings

Pathway to health

Many digestive disorders, such as indigestion, ulcers and irritable bowel syndrome, may be aggravated by stress or deficiencies in the immune system. T'ai chi, the Chinese movement and meditation therapy, is thought to both cure and prevent such problems, especially stress. T'ai chi may also enhance the efficiency of the immune system by increasing the rate and flow of lymphatic fluid.

USING THE 12345+ FOOD PLAN
Australian nutritionists have developed an alternative easy-to-remember food guide. For each day, it suggests one serving of meat or alternatives such as pulses, two servings of milk and milk products, three servings of fruits, four servings of vegetables and five servings of bread and cereals, plus a very small portion of whatever else you fancy.

As food travels, several organs – stomach, liver, pancreas and the intestine, in addition to the salivary glands – add digestive juices and other substances to it that help to break the food down into simpler substances. Once the foods are broken down, or digested, the smallest units (nutrients and many non-nutrients) are absorbed through the linings of the digestive organs into the bloodstream and the lymphatic system, which distribute them throughout the body. Waste materials remaining after digestion are expelled from the body as urine or faeces.

BALANCING YOUR DIET

Doctors and nutrition experts tell you to eat a 'balanced' diet, but this does not mean eating the same amount of each type of food. You need to eat more of some foods than others to meet your body's needs.

For a balanced diet, the variety of foods you eat should work in harmony with one another. Over the years, nutrition experts have drawn charts and plotted graphs to help people visualise which foods should be eaten in larger, or smaller, quantities. As more has been learned about nutrition, the

diagrams have changed accordingly. Once food groups were shown as sections in a pie-chart; today, the pyramid is a popular, more representative shape.

Children, pregnant women, breastfeeding mothers and sick or elderly people may require foods in different proportions, but for most people the following guidelines are appropriate for a well-balanced diet.

The highest number of servings should come from complex-carbohydrate foods, the wholemeal varieties of bread, cereals, and pasta, brown rice and jacket potatoes. Bear in mind, however, that these foods are better for you if they are eaten with very little or no butter or rich sauces because these add many calories but few nutrients.

A large number of food portions should consist of vegetables, eaten either raw or lightly cooked. After that, try to eat almost as many portions of fruits. This will provide a wide array of vitamins and minerals.

Meat and dairy products, such as cheese and yoghurt, are important sources of proteins. They are often high in fat, however, so you should limit your intake of these foods to one or two small servings each day.

The higher the fat content of foods, the less you need of them. Fats appear at the top of the food pyramid as a way of demonstrating how little you should eat each day in comparison with other types of foods. Products high in refined sugars also appear at the top, indicating that they are desirable only as a very small part of your diet.

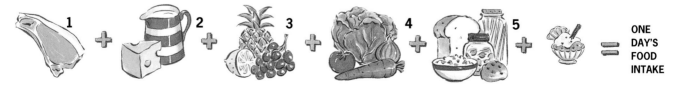

1 + **2** + **3** + **4** + **5** + = ONE DAY'S FOOD INTAKE

What is a portion of food?

Being able roughly to judge food portions, or serving sizes, is an important part of controlling your weight and maintaining a balanced diet. The portions listed in diet books and nutrition guides usually weigh between 85 and 100 grams (3 to 3½ ounces). Sometimes, food portions are listed in tablespoonfuls (tbsp), where one tablespoon is 15 millilitres.

To help you recognise food portions, take a dinner plate (one you use every day) and, using kitchen scales and a tablespoon, serve out different foods. Look at how much space they fill on your plate. You may discover that your food likes and dislikes affect the size you think a portion should be.

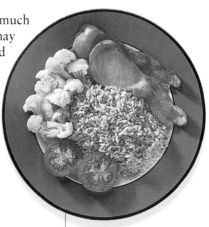

RECOGNISING FOOD PORTIONS
Each of these foods is a portion:
50 grams (1¼ ounces) of cauliflower,
a medium-size tomato, 200 grams
(7 ounces) of cooked rice, and two
rashers of bacon.

COMMON FOOD PORTIONS

DAIRY PRODUCTS	WEIGHT	CALORIES	PROTEIN grams	FAT grams	CARBOHYDRATE grams
Cheddar cheese	25 g (1 oz)	124	8	10	trace
Yoghurt (low-fat) fruit-flavoured	115 g (4 oz)	104	4	1	20
Yoghurt (low-fat) plain	115 g (4 oz)	65	6	1	9
CEREALS					
Bread (2 medium slices) wholemeal	70 g (2½ oz)	153	6	1.8	29
Bread roll or bap (1 roll) wholemeal	75 g (2¾ oz)	193	7	2	39
Cornflakes (no milk)	25 g (1 oz)	108	2.5	0.2	26
MEAT					
Lamb chops (loin) grilled, lean (2)	175 g (6 oz)	207	26	11.5	0
Burger (beef) fried (2)	85 g (3 oz)	224	17	15	0.6
Turkey (light meat, no skin) roast	115 g (4 oz)	152	34	1.8	0
Beef (round tip, lean) roast	115 g (4 oz)	259	32	14.5	0
Pork (leg, lean) roast	115 g (4 oz)	213	35	7.9	0
FISH					
Sardines (canned in brine)	115 g (4 oz)	198	25	11	0
Trout (baked)	115 g (4 oz)	155	27	5	0
Haddock (steamed)	115 g (4 oz)	116	27	1	0
Salmon (poached)	115 g (4 oz)	227	23	15	0
FRUITS					
Apple	115 g (4 oz)	54	0.4	0	14
Banana	125 g (4½ oz)	123	1.5	0.3	30
Pears (fresh)	140 g (5 oz)	56	0.4	0	14
Pears (canned in juice)	125 g (4½ oz)	43	0.4	0	11
VEGETABLES – RAW					
Cabbage	50 g (1¾ oz)	13	1	trace	2.1
Carrots, grated	50 g (1¾ oz)	18	0.3	trace	3.9
Cauliflower	50 g (1¾ oz)	17	2	trace	1.5
Broccoli	50 g (1¾ oz)	17	2	trace	0.9
Spinach	50 g (1¾ oz)	13	2	trace	0.8
VEGETABLES – COOKED					
Cabbage	100 g (3½ oz)	14	1	0	2
Carrots, boiled	100 g (3½ oz)	24	0.6	0	5
Cauliflower	100 g (3½ oz)	28	3	1	2
Broccoli	100 g (3½ oz)	24	3	1	1
Spinach	100 g (3½ oz)	19	2	1	1

Hidden extras

When helping yourself to food, try to remember that equal-sized portions do not contain the same quantity of food energy. The number of calories in a 115 gram (4 ounce) portion of chips (280) and a similar portion of boiled spinach (33) are very different.

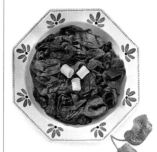

ADDING EXTRA CALORIES
Spinach is low in calories but adding butter raises its calorie count substantially. Calories listed for a portion do not include toppings. For example, a portion of beef does not include gravy.

The Nutritionist

Nutritionists ask people about their eating patterns and other aspects of their lives. They then give advice on how to modify the diet to achieve better health, or make improvements to help treat a medical condition.

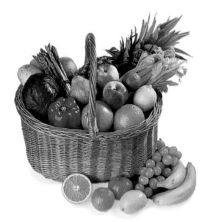

NATURAL GOODNESS
In line with current dietary guidelines, nutritionists recommend that you eat at least five servings of fruits and vegetables a day.

CONSULTING A NUTRITIONIST
Many people see nutritionists to get advice about a medical condition, for example diabetes. Others may simply want to eat a better diet to improve their overall health.

A nutritionist will discuss any nutritional worries or problems that affect your everyday eating habits. He or she will assess your current eating pattern and check for any dietary deficiency or imbalance and will then be able to advise you on how to improve your diet. If you have a special condition – for example, if you are pregnant or have heart disease, or you want to lose or gain weight – a nutritionist can recommend modifications to your diet.

What happens on the first visit to a nutritionist?

A nutritionist will ask you about your objectives (whether they are to treat a particular complaint such as heart disease or to lose weight, for example), your health and your current diet. She will discuss your lifestyle, your eating pattern, any allergies you may have, and any restrictions that you have placed on your diet – if you are a committed vegetarian, for instance.

A nutritionist may also ask you about any digestive problems and about your likes and dislikes concerning food. You will probably be asked to keep a food diary for a few days after your first visit. This will be discussed on your next visit. If your aim is to lose or gain weight, the nutritionist may record your weight, percentage of body fat and measurements (chest, waist and hips).

What is a food diary?

A food diary is one of the best ways to find out what you are really taking in. When keeping a food diary, you will write down the exact amounts of everything you eat and drink for about three to seven days (including every cup of tea and biscuit).

Using the completed diary, the nutritionist will be able to analyse your diet, compare your intake with the recommended values, check for any deficiencies – in folic acid, iron or calcium, for example – and then advise you on specific changes that you should make (see also p. 14).

Will the nutritionist perform any tests?

If your diet lacks a particular nutrient and the nutritionist suspects that you are suffering deficiency symptoms, she should consult your doctor. The nutritionist will describe the deficiency and suggest that you have a test – for example, a blood test for anaemia, which might be caused by lack of iron in your diet.

Will the nutritionist recommend recipe ideas?

Yes. Your food diary will reveal whether your diet is unbalanced or if you have erratic eating habits. If the diary indicates that you are often too busy to prepare proper meals – you may skip breakfast and eat too many snack meals – the nutritionist will suggest quick, nourishing recipes using foods you enjoy that you can prepare at home.

If you are a vegetarian, the nutritionist will suggest various ways of mixing beans and grains and other foods to get the right quality of proteins. The nutritionist will check your food diary for sources of iron and how often you eat them.

If there is a deficiency, the nutritionist will give you recipes that use iron-rich foods, such as cereals, dark green leafy vegetables and egg yolks. The nutritionist will also tell you how to mix iron-rich foods with foods rich in vitamin C to increase iron absorption – for example, by eating your breakfast cereal with fresh strawberries.

How soon will my new eating habits have an effect on the way I look and feel?

This will depend on what sort of changes you need to make and how soon you can put them into practice. Most people start to feel and see an improvement in two or three weeks. If you are aiming to lose weight, you should lose between one to two pounds per week – any more may be dangerous – and, therefore, you should see a noticeable difference after two or three weeks.

LOW-FAT COOKING

A nutritionist can suggest ways of satisfying your taste for sweet foods while cutting down on fat.

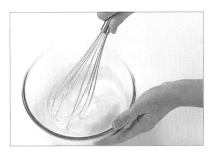

1 *Whisk 3 eggs and 40 g (1½ oz) caster sugar until thick. Fold in 70 g (2½ oz) sieved flour, then 1 tbsp skimmed milk and 1 tsp grated lemon rind. Spoon into an 18 cm (7 in) cake tin and bake at 180°C (350°F, Gas 4) for 20 minutes until risen.*

He or she may recommend a recipe for a low-fat cake with a nutritious topping like the one shown below.

2 *Let cool. Slice in half, fill with low-fat yoghurt and fruit. Spread more yoghurt and fruit on top.*

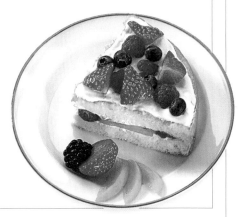

How often do nutritionists see their patients?

Sometimes a single visit is sufficient to discuss the patient's main problems and provide enough advice to achieve the nutritional goals. At least one or two follow-up consultations may be needed to monitor progress and set further targets. Seeing the nutritionist more than once will help to keep you motivated.

WHAT YOU CAN DO AT HOME

To motivate yourself, write down your nutritional goals and objectives. For example, 'I want to feel more energetic and healthy' or 'I want to lose seven pounds'. Also, keep a diary of everything you eat and drink for three days, more if you can manage it. Analyse your food diary to work out your good and bad eating habits.

▶ *Look at the timing of your meals. Do you eat breakfast? Do you eat at regular intervals during the day? Do you skip meals? These are important questions. Do you eat very little during the day but a very big meal in the evening? This eating pattern is far from ideal.*

▶ *Look at what kinds and amounts of food you eat. Large quantities of high-fat foods – for example, pastry dishes – are undesirable, while eating five portions of fruit and vegetables a day is good.*

▶ *Then look at the way your diet is balanced. Eating the same foods day after day is not good for you, while eating a wide variety of foods will keep you healthy.*

▶ *Write down some easy changes you can make. For instance, start eating breakfast. Do not skip meals. Eat fruit instead of chocolate. Aim to make just one change at a time.*

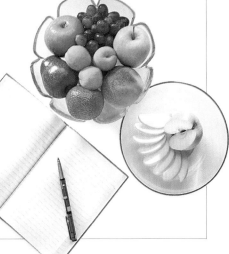

KEEPING YOUR BODY FUELLED

Regardless of physical activity, your body uses up to 70 per cent of its daily energy expenditure simply by keeping organs working, replacing cells, repairing damage and building tissue.

Are snacks harmful?
Sometimes a snack is what you need to keep you going, but try to keep your total diet in mind, and give some thought to the number of calories and amount of fat you are eating.

  Snack foods, such as crisps, chips and nuts, all contain high amounts of fat and are high in calories. Eat them only occasionally. If you want a snack, choose fruit, wholemeal biscuits or perhaps some fresh vegetables dipped in a low-fat sauce.

Foods have different energy, or caloric, values because they contain varying combinations and amounts of protein, fat, carbohydrate and water. For example, a 50 gram (1¾ ounce) serving of cauliflower supplies only seven calories while a wholemeal roll of the same weight provides 135.

MEASURING FOOD ENERGY
The energy in the foods you eat is measured in units called calories, which is the energy needed to raise the temperature of one millilitre of water by 1° Centigrade. But since this is so small, health and nutrition professionals usually speak of calories in units of 1000, called a kilocalorie or Calorie (with a capital 'C'). These measurements are usually abbreviated as kcal or cal. You may sometimes see a reference to a kilojoule. This refers to an even smaller unit of calories: 4.18 kilojoules equal one calorie.

  Basic nutrients differ in their energy content. A gram of either pure carbohydrate or protein contains four calories. A gram of pure fat, however, contains nine, while a gram of water has no caloric value. The caloric value of a food only indicates its energy level and does not describe the proportion of other nutrients, such as protein, carbohydrates, vitamins and minerals. Therefore, if a food is high in calories it is not necessarily high in all nutrients.

  Everybody needs a certain amount of energy from food simply to maintain basic bodily functions such as breathing, blood circulation and body temperature when the body is at rest. This is called the basal metabolic rate (BMR). Further calories are necessary for the body to be active. The number of calories each individual requires varies enormously, depending on age, sex, size and metabolic rate. For example, a sedentary woman aged 65 years weighing about 54.5 kilograms (120 pounds) burns about 1500 calories a day whereas an active 25-year-old active woman weighing the same requires about 2000 calories to fuel her body.

FOODS CONTAINING APPROXIMATELY 1000 CALORIES

2 bars dark chocolate (100 g/3½ oz each)
3 packets of peanuts (175 g/6 oz)
3 (420 g/15 oz) cans baked beans
4 regular portions fast-food chips
7 sausages (standard size)
8 (350 ml/12 fl oz) cans of cola
12 slices white bread
11 glasses of wine (125 ml/4½ fl oz each)
15 large glasses skimmed milk
16 bananas
30 slices of ham
85 boiled carrots
250 servings of lettuce (¼ head each)
700 g (25 oz) of roast chicken (white meat)

WHICH IS MORE FATTENING?
The number of calories in food can vary enormously. Both 95 tomatoes and two ¼ pound cheeseburgers supply 1000 calories.

At certain times, a person's basal metabolic rate may change and consequently calorie need is affected. During periods of illness or stress, the basal metabolic rate tends to slow down and fewer calories will be needed, but during pregnancy and while breastfeeding it speeds up. A pregnant woman needs about 300 calories more a day and a nursing mother an extra 500 calories.

Active people expend much more energy than sedentary individuals. Walking and gardening are two common activities that increase your body's energy needs. A man who drives to work, has a sedentary job and spends most of his leisure time watching television will only need about 2200 calories, while an athlete in training burns up about 4000 to 5000 calories per day.

MAINTAINING BODY WEIGHT

Balancing the amount of energy you consume with the amount you expend is vital if you want to maintain your ideal body weight. If your diet is providing more calories than are being burned by your daily activities, the remainder will be stored by your body as fat, which may lead to obesity. But if your food intake is not fulfilling your energy requirements, your body will turn to any fat stored in tissues. If that becomes depleted, it will begin to break down muscle tissue, including cardiac muscle.

Your scales are the best indicator of whether you are eating too much or just enough. Weight gain or loss depends on how many calories are in the total diet, not necessarily on the particular foods you eat. It may be worth cutting down on some foods high in refined sugar, however, since the bulk of their calories are 'empty' (calories without nutritional value).

DO YOU NEED THREE
MEALS A DAY?

How many meals you have each day depends on your activity level and personal preference. Some people feel and work best on four or five small meals.

Obtaining a carbohydrate boost mid morning and afternoon by eating a piece of fruit, for example, can help to maintain blood sugar levels and stop you feeling tired. It is thought that eating a big breakfast, less lunch and a very small supper will aid digestion. In other words, you should breakfast like a king, lunch like a prince and

AGE AND ENERGY REQUIREMENTS

A five or six-year-old child requires about the same number of calories per day as his or her 75-year-old grandmother, despite the differences in their weight and size. This is because their bodies are using energy in different ways. The child needs a lot of energy for growth and development; the mature adult, however, is likely to be fairly inactive, and needs the energy primarily for maintaining bodily processes.

AGE	ACTIVITY LEVELS	ENERGY REQUIRED
INFANT		
Less than one year		950 kcals
CHILD		
4–6 years		1710 kcals
BOYS		
11–14 years		2220 kcals
GIRLS		
11–14 years		1845 kcals
MEN		
18–34 years	Sedentary	2510 kcals
	Active	2900 kcals
	Very Active	3350 kcals
35–64 years	Sedentary	2400 kcals
	Active	2750 kcals
	Very Active	3350 kcals
65–74 years	Sedentary	2330 kcals
75+ years	Sedentary	2100 kcals
WOMEN		
18–54 years	Sedentary	1940 kcals
	Active	2150 kcals
	Very Active	2500 kcals
	Pregnant	2400 kcals
	Breastfeeding	2750 kcals
55–74 years	Sedentary	1900 kcals
	Active	2000 kcals
75+ years	Sedentary	1810 kcals

dine like a pauper. This allows the digestive system to break down food during the active part of the day and give you a steady supply of nutrients. If you eat a heavy meal during the evening, it may not be digested properly and may cause indigestion.

Solving a

Dietary Imbalance

Serious but rare illnesses such as scurvy and beriberi are caused by food deficiencies or dietary imbalance. A range of more common but less serious complaints can also be caused by deficiencies in your diet, but these can be easily adjusted.

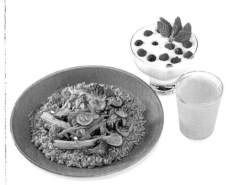

FOODS TO PREVENT ANAEMIA
Exhaustion and shortness of breath may be due to anaemia, which can result if you are not eating enough foods containing iron. Animal products such as fish and red meat are the best sources. Green vegetables are good sources but need to be consumed with vitamin C, for example, by drinking orange juice with your meal.

Feeling lethargic and run down does not necessarily mean that you are ill, but it can have a profound effect on your day-to-day life. The causes of these symptoms are diverse: you may not be taking enough exercise, you may not be getting enough sleep or you may be suffering from anxiety. Or, you may be eating the wrong kinds of food. Excessive amounts of sugary foods, such as cakes and biscuits, or of sweetened drinks such as colas, produce a temporary sugar-high but in the long term your energy levels will be greatly reduced.

Another food-related problem, a common digestive complaint, is constipation. This is often caused by a lack of dietary fibre. So be sure to eat plenty of wholewheat breads and cereals, dried beans and peas and fresh fruit and vegetables.

FOODS TO ALLEVIATE CONSTIPATION
An inability to pass stools can be the result of eating too many refined foods and not enough fibre. Eating unprocessed wheat bran makes faeces bulkier and stimulates bowel function.

CURING MINOR HEALTH PROBLEMS

Below are some common health problems caused by a lack of specific nutrients in the diet and some recommended foods to help alleviate the symptoms. There can be other causes for each of these conditions, however, so adapting your diet may solve only part of the problem. If symptoms persist, consult your doctor.

Add a tablespoonful of bran to breakfast cereal or other foods once a day

PROBLEM	POSSIBLE DEFICIENCY	EAT MORE
MOUTH		
Bleeding gums.	Vitamin C.	Citrus fruit, sweet peppers, potatoes.
Sore tongue, cracked corners, recurrent ulcers, cracked/dry lips.	Vitamins B_{12}, B_2, B_6, folic acid.	Yeast extract, potatoes pork, milk, spinach, fortified breakfast cereal.
SKIN		
Dry and rough skin.	Vitamins A, B_2, E, essential fatty acids.	Milk, dark green and orange vegetables, most vegetable oils, fish.
HAIR		
Poor growth, dry.	Vitamin A, zinc, essential fatty acids.	Milk, dark green and orange vegetables, oily fish.
NAILS		
Thinning; flattened and concave or spoon-shaped appearance.	Iron.	Red meat, wholemeal bread, spinach.

Why breakfast is so important

While you sleep, your body is on a mini fast, and blood sugar levels are low. A breakfast of complex carbohydrates in the form of unrefined cereals or wholemeal bread will recharge blood sugar levels and provide the energy you need until lunch time.

Choosing a varied diet

Normally, during the course of the day, the foods people eat come from more than one food group. If you eat cereal and fruit for breakfast, soup and a sandwich for lunch, and fish or meat, potatoes and vegetables for the main meal, you will have achieved a healthy and varied diet. But most people find it impossible to eat a balanced diet every day. Special occasions, vacations, illness or pressures of work can all play havoc with your diet.

But do not let food become an obsession. The secret of a good diet is not to count your calories but to eat the right balance of foods over a period of three or four days. If you overindulge in chocolate one day, spend the next couple of days following a diet that is low in fat and rich in vegetables and fruit, while avoiding sugary desserts.

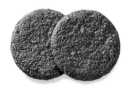

SATISFYING SNACK
Two wholewheat biscuits provide 140 calories but they also offer fibre.

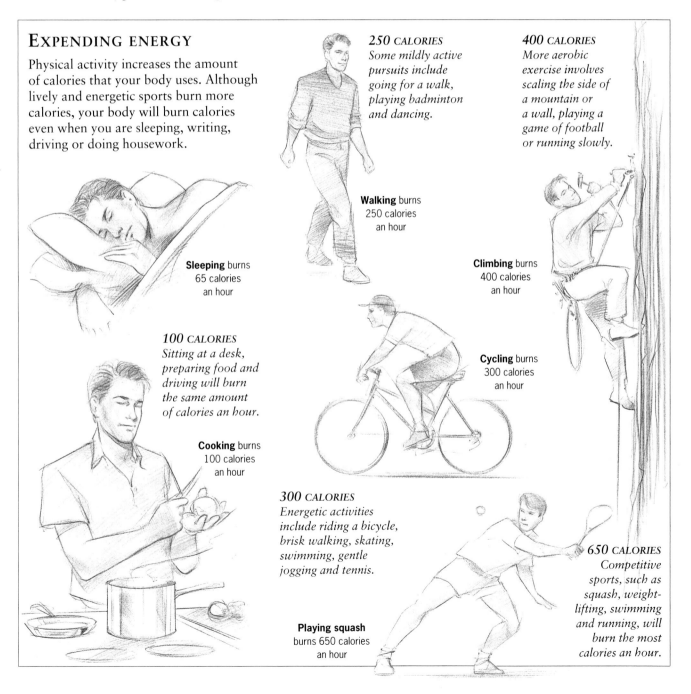

EXPENDING ENERGY

Physical activity increases the amount of calories that your body uses. Although lively and energetic sports burn more calories, your body will burn calories even when you are sleeping, writing, driving or doing housework.

Sleeping burns 65 calories an hour

100 CALORIES
Sitting at a desk, preparing food and driving will burn the same amount of calories an hour.

Cooking burns 100 calories an hour

250 CALORIES
Some mildly active pursuits include going for a walk, playing badminton and dancing.

Walking burns 250 calories an hour

Cycling burns 300 calories an hour

300 CALORIES
Energetic activities include riding a bicycle, brisk walking, skating, swimming, gentle jogging and tennis.

Playing squash burns 650 calories an hour

400 CALORIES
More aerobic exercise involves scaling the side of a mountain or a wall, playing a game of football or running slowly.

Climbing burns 400 calories an hour

650 CALORIES
Competitive sports, such as squash, weightlifting, swimming and running, will burn the most calories an hour.

The Busy Family

Feeding a family is not easy. However hard you try, there are always the pressures of too little time, dissimilar food preferences, and the constant temptation to substitute less nutritious fast foods for home-cooked meals. The result can be a poor diet that causes health problems. The solution to this problem, however, does not mean sacrificing variety or favourite family meals.

Sandra Merton and her husband, Eddie, have two school-age children. Anticipating future college costs, Sandra took a job at the local nursing home six months ago, working on the early morning shift. Since she started, she has noticed that the family's eating habits have become unhealthy.

Eleven-year-old Charlie eats nothing but hamburgers, chips, colas and sweets. He will not eat vegetables nor, except for the occasional banana, fruit. Sandra suspects Charlie is not eating the breakfast she leaves for him. She is worried that he seems to be developing acne. Fifteen-year-old Maggie tends to skip breakfast and eats as little as possible at the table, although Sandra catches her taking snacks from the refrigerator while they watch television in the evening. Lately, Maggie's hair has looked dull and dry. Both children have school meals, but the foods they choose seem to be of the fast food variety – pizzas, burgers and tacos.

To help care for the children when Sandra is at work, Eddie switched to a night job. He is asleep when the children eat their breakfast, but supervises their after-school activities. He shops for food when the refrigerator seems empty but his food choices are haphazard. Since they began their new schedule, Eddie has gained weight, which Sandra believes is a result of his snacking on crisps instead of eating a proper meal during the day. At work, he buys a sandwich and soft drink from the canteen and eats chocolate bars when he gets hungry.

During the week, Sandra arrives home from work at two-thirty, and Eddie leaves at six in the evening. Sandra and the children eat their evening meal while watching television. Because her job makes her tired, Sandra often does not have the energy to cook so they often rely on takeaways. The Mertons usually eat together only at the weekends, but the meals are quite stressful, because during them Eddie and Sandra quiz the children about their school work.

IRREGULAR HOURS
Shift-work disrupts normal eating patterns and very often means people feel hungry at times when a wholesome meal is not available.

TIME SAVING
When family members eat at different times, frequently they will opt for easily prepared processed foods. They consider the only meals worth taking trouble over are for the whole family.

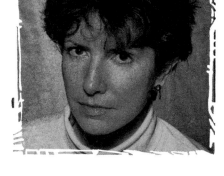

FINANCE
A diet of fast foods, snacks and takeaways is expensive, costing more than foods prepared at home.

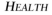

HEALTH
Irregular eating habits create health problems because they make it difficult to achieve a balanced diet.

COMMUNICATION
Finding time to share ideas and information can be difficult for a busy family. When communication takes place only at meal times, tension and disagreements can make eating together stressful.

WHAT SHOULD THE MERTONS DO?

Sandra knows it is necessary to get every member of the family involved in changing their eating habits. Without cooperation, little progress will be made and the eating situation will deteriorate further, harming everyone's health and appearance.

Since Saturday is a day when the whole family is free, Sandra should get them together to discuss her concerns. Before the meeting, she should make a list of their diet and health problems and how she thinks they can be solved. The family should agree to set aside one hour each week to discuss meal plans.

As a first step, Sandra should get everyone to take part in choosing the foods they eat, with an emphasis on good health.

Eddie must realise that he has to lose weight – he has gained 6.8 kilograms (15 pounds) since he started on the night shift. He has to give up his unhealthy snacks, especially during the day. He should also find out what forms of exercise he can do during his free time.

Both children must learn to alter their eating habits – Charlie to a less 'high-fried/sugar' diet and Maggie to a diet that is much more balanced.

Meals need to be made into a more relaxed occasion and discussions about school work should be saved for other times.

Action Plan

IRREGULAR HOURS
Help Eddie to make a list of tasty, healthful foods he could prepare for himself after he returns home from work and during the day. Substitute low-calorie snacks, such as fruit, for the chocolate eaten during working hours.

FINANCE
Collect the bills for food purchased over a four-week period, and add up how much was spent on various items. Draft a food budget and an eating plan that provides a balanced diet – and is cheaper as well.

HEALTH
Make a list of all the health problems and conditions the family faces because of poor dietary habits. Also make a list of healthful foods that will help the family to avoid vitamin and mineral deficiencies. Begin looking for interesting ways to incorporate these items into the family's new eating plan.

COMMUNICATION
Reserve family mealtimes for listening to the children and discuss pleasant and noncontroversial topics. Let the children have their say when shopping and cooking the family's meals. Having greater control will make them more interested in the foods they eat.

TIME SAVING
When preparing meals at the weekend, make extra and freeze in portion-size containers. (Portions of food can be microwaved quickly and easily when Eddie is by himself during the day; Sandra and the children can do the same later in the evening.)

HOW THINGS TURNED OUT FOR THE MERTONS

The Merton family meetings were successful for the first three weeks, but then the children became bored and restless, so they were cut down to 30 minutes.

Sandra and Eddie set a food budget for the month and a limit on takeaway food to once a week. However, takeaways still figure in at least two meals a week and the budget has not yet been met. But substantial savings are being made and are being put aside for the college fund.

Eddie finds it hard to break his snack habit during the day, so every time he gets hungry he takes a brisk walk. When shopping for food, he tries to resist buying unhealthy snack fare; he now buys more fresh fruit and vegetables.

The Saturday shopping trip is now being done on a rota system, with either Maggie or Charlie accompanying one of their parents. This has made both children more food conscious, which has had a knock-on effect on some of their

school meals; they no longer consist solely of fast foods. With Charlie's help, Maggie has started to select recipes for her mother to make. She now spends some of her time reading about health and beauty as well as pop stars.

After a month, Sandra told everyone she wanted them all to take turns making the evening meal. She knew the family had turned the corner when Charlie volunteered to cook the roast meat and potatoes for Sunday lunch.

THE EFFECTS OF CULTURE ON EATING

There are many things that influence your choice of food and these are quite irrespective of nutritional value. Identifying what they are may change your attitudes towards the food you eat.

Savouring the flavour
French children learn how to use their sense of taste in school. Part of their curriculum involves identifying and describing the tastes of saltiness, bitterness, sweetness and sourness, followed by exercises in which food textures are explored. Finally, the children learn how to describe blends of flavours and textures in specific foods.

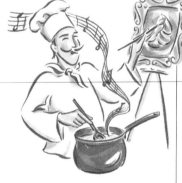

REFINED TASTE
The French believe that, like a fine painting or a piece of classical music, the artistry of a cook and the quality of a meal may be appreciated fully only when the eater's sense of taste has been educated.

Much more than flavour or food values influence our decision about what to eat. Cultural background may make food that is acceptable in one country, for instance, horse meat in France, anathema in others, such as in the animal-loving United Kingdom.

Political beliefs may alter eating habits. The low pay and poor treatment of grape pickers on the west coast of the United States spurred Cesar Chavez (1927–94) to lead a successful embargo against the fruit in California during the 1960s. Another consideration is religion. Jews and Muslims never eat pork since the pig is regarded as unclean, but this prohibition may have its origins in a caution about eating meat that can cause disease if undercooked.

Subliminal desires

Food and drink manufacturers often use subtle means to persuade you to choose their products. For example, when watching movies and television dramas, if you see

THE IDEAL SHAPE

Fashion usually features models who are thin because designers claim clothes hang better on them. Many women regard this thinness as worthy of being emulated. In attempting to achieve this 'ideal' body shape, they often regard food as the enemy. In fact, food in the form of a balanced diet is the best friend your body has.

a can of cola in the hero's hand it is unlikely to be there by chance. Companies pay a lot of money to advertise in this way – it is what the advertising industry calls product placement. Their hope is that the next time you buy a canned drink, although the image you have seen may not come to mind, it may have had a subconscious influence on your choice of product.

SYMBOLISM, FESTIVALS AND CELEBRATIONS

Food plays a prominent role in many of society's rituals, particularly festivals and celebrations; it even features at funerals. Food is often used as a sign of love and friendship. Sweets, for example, are associated with comfort and security; chocolates are given to friends and relatives as a sign of affection and are a particularly popular Valentine's Day gift.

Many foods are traditionally eaten at certain festivals and celebrations. Eggs, for example, symbolise Easter in many

parts of the world, while roast turkey is eaten at Christmas in Britain and at Thanksgiving in the United States.

Many occasions are incomplete without a cake. Cakes are eaten at birthday parties, christenings and weddings. The tiered cake is the focal point of most wedding celebrations, with the cutting of the cake being a time-honoured tradition. A layer of wedding cake is often saved to be eaten at the first anniversary or at the christening of the couple's first baby.

CHAPTER 2

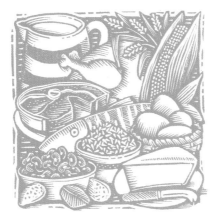

THE POWER
OF PROTEIN

*Proteins are essential constituents of
all human cells, controlling such vital processes
as metabolism and providing the structural basis
of many body tissues, such as muscles and skin.
They enable the body to grow and repair itself,
and they play a role in protecting the body against
infection. Protein-rich foods are mainly of animal
origin – meat, fish, poultry, eggs and milk.
But some protein is also present in wheat,
rice, corn, nuts, peas, beans and lentils.*

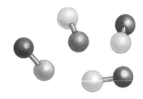

Proteins in food are long chains of amino acids that are broken down during digestion

Polypeptides, which are the next stage in protein digestion, are shorter chains

Peptides are chains with even fewer links, which then break down into constituent amino acids

Individual amino acids are finally reassembled into the new proteins that are needed by the body

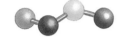

BREAKING DOWN AND REASSEMBLING PROTEIN
The proteins that are used by body cells differ from those found in foods, although both types consist of the same amino acids. After ingestion, the amino acids in foods are rearranged into the protein structures needed by the body.

PROTEIN FOR LIFE

Proteins are vital for growth and health and form part of many of the foods we eat. Some foods, however, have to be eaten with others to provide the quality of protein the body needs.

Individual proteins are made up of various combinations of at least 50, and up to several thousand, amino acids strung together in a long chain. A complete protein depends upon this chain of amino acids gathering into a highly complex, multi-layered string, and then going on to twist itself into intricate three-dimensional shapes. Proteins can be made by the body internally as well as imported ready-made via the diet. The important function of the dietary proteins is their supply of constituent amino acids, which the body can resynthesise into new specialised proteins tailored for its various vital processes.

Amino acids come in 22 different forms and all are needed to build the many different kinds of proteins the body requires. Eight of these amino acids (ten for children) fall into the category termed essential amino acids – this means that they have to

be supplied in food because the body is unable to manufacture them. Without them, the body cannot build the full range of proteins in amounts that are necessary for the growth and maintenance of the various tissues. The remaining 14 amino acids are called non-essential amino acids because the body is able to synthesise them itself. But despite their name, non-essential amino acids are just as important for health as the essential ones because all proteins are constructed from arrangements of both essential and non-essential amino acids.

HOW THE BODY USES PROTEIN

The enzymes in the digestive system break down the protein in food into its constituent amino acids, which then circulate in the bloodstream. The body cells stack up the amino acids like building blocks according to which amino acids the cell

FOOD PROTEIN QUALITY

A food's protein quality is determined by the amounts of essential amino acids that it contains. Eggs are the best source of

protein – they have a maximum score of 100. This chart shows the protein quality of foods as measured against the egg.

HIGH AND LOW QUALITY PROTEIN
Animal foods, such as fish and meat, provide the body with sufficient essential amino acids. Plant foods, on the other hand, lack one or more of the essential amino acids and therefore have a poor protein quality. When cereals and beans are eaten together, however, they complement each other to provide a higher quality – and more complete – protein.

PROTEIN SOURCE	PROTEIN QUALITY
Egg	100
Fish	90
Meat	80
Cow's milk	80
Grain with pulses (peas or lentils)	80
Soya beans	75
Oatmeal	65
Rice	57
Peas	48
Lentils	45
Kidney beans	44
Wholegrain bread	40

CAUTION

If the carbohydrates and fats in a diet are not supplying sufficient calories – for instance, when an individual is on a strict diet or suffering from malnutrition – the body will burn protein instead. Using protein as a fuel may not leave enough for its primary function of cell production.

needs. Each amino acid has a unique role, and another one cannot be used in its place, so it is important to make sure your diet is varied enough to provide all the amino acids that your body needs.

COMPLETE AND INCOMPLETE PROTEINS

Proteins vary greatly in the number, type and arrangement of their amino acids, and so do their quality or 'biological value'.

Animal foods are a major source of protein and the protein present in meat, fish, eggs, milk and milk products contains all the essential amino acids in the proportions the body requires. Animal protein, therefore, is known as 'complete' protein.

The protein in plant foods – cereals (grain products), nuts and pulses (peas, beans and lentils) – also contributes differ-

ent amounts and types of essential amino acids. However, unlike animal sources, no single plant source is able to provide a full complement of essential amino acids. Plant proteins, therefore, are 'incomplete' and have a low 'biological value'.

In order for plant foods to supply complete proteins, those that are low in certain essential amino acids should be eaten with those that are relatively high in those amino acids. Wheat, corn and rice, for example, contain plenty of the essential amino acid methionine but not very much of another amino acid called lysine, whereas beans contain a good supply of lysine but not much methionine. Without knowing the chemical and biological reasons, cooks around the world for centuries have combined grains and pulses to provide complete protein in a single dish – for example, baked beans on toast.

How much protein is enough?

The body gains and loses protein every day – for instance, simply cutting your nails or hair will cause a minor loss of protein, whereas every four days one-half of the intestinal lining, which has a vast surface area, is replaced. Therefore, it is important to have some protein every day to replace the worn-out tissues that result from general bodily wear and tear and to manufacture new blood cells, hormones and enzymes.

Bodily proteins

There are two distinct types of protein in the body – insoluble structural proteins that are basically fibrous in form, and physiologically active soluble proteins, which have a globular structure.

The fibrous type includes such proteins as keratin in hair and nails, myosin in muscle tissue, collagen in connective tissues such as skin, tendons and cartilage, and fibrin found in scar tissue.

The physiologically active class of protein includes most of the enzymes involved in the metabolic activities of the body. This type of protein also includes a number of hormones, for example insulin and prolactin (milk secretion), haemoglobin, which transports oxygen in the blood, and the antibodies used in the body's defence system.

COMPLEMENTARY PROTEINS

Complementary protein food sources do not need to be eaten at the same meal, but they do need to be eaten at the next meal on the same day. This is because the body stores essential amino acids for only a few hours.

MATCHING YOUR PROTEIN FOODS
The solid red line in this diagram shows the better combination of plant foods to obtain quality protein. The broken green line shows the combination that does not always provide complete protein.

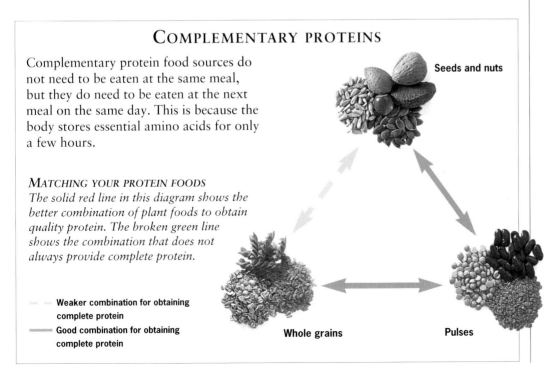

Seeds and nuts

Whole grains

Pulses

- - - Weaker combination for obtaining complete protein
—— Good combination for obtaining complete protein

RECOMMENDED DAILY INTAKE OF PROTEIN

The amount of protein you need to consume will vary throughout your life. Pregnant women need an extra six grams of protein per day. Mothers who are breast-feeding need an extra 11 grams.

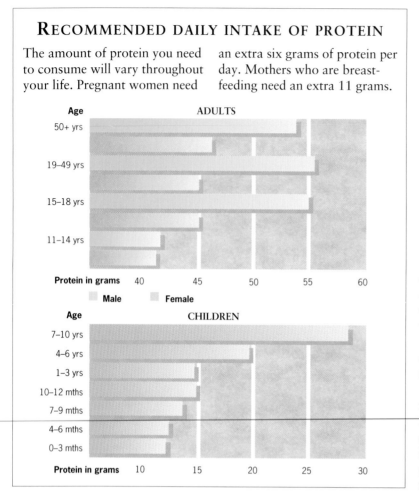

ADULTS

Age	Protein in grams	40	45	50	55	60
50+ yrs						
19–49 yrs						
15–18 yrs						
11–14 yrs						

Male Female

CHILDREN

Age	Protein in grams	10	15	20	25	30
7–10 yrs						
4–6 yrs						
1–3 yrs						
10–12 mths						
7–9 mths						
4–6 mths						
0–3 mths						

An individual's protein requirements are often calculated according to body weight: 0.75 grams of protein per kilogram of body weight is considered enough for a healthy adult. (To convert your weight from pounds to kilograms, divide it by 2.3.) If, for example, you weigh 55 kilograms then multiply 0.75 by 55. This result is 41.25 grams – your average protein need per day.

A well-balanced diet should easily provide enough protein since it is available in such a wide range of foods. Between 10 and 15 per cent of the total calories in your diet should come from protein. An average-sized, middle-aged man, for example, could easily fulfill his daily protein need with a cheese sandwich, a glass of milk, one serving of chicken breast, and one portion each of potatoes and peas. On the other hand, a woman in her sixties would only need a 115 grams (4 ounces) of yoghurt, an egg, a glass of milk, a small serving of fish, some rice and three wholemeal biscuits.

At various times in life, however, people need extra protein. Pregnant and breast-feeding women need to ensure they have an adequate intake. But too much protein during pregnancy is undesirable, and taking protein supplements may lead to complications. People suffering from a severe injury,

PICK A PORTION OF PROTEIN

Illustrated below are the amounts of protein in high-protein foods like meat, fish and milk. Another food that is rich in complete protein is eggs (see p. 30).

Also shown are the amounts of protein in plant foods. Because the amino acids in plant foods are incomplete, they need to be complemented as shown on page 31.

Baked beans 115 g (4 oz) incomplete

Chicken without skin, 25 g (1 oz)

Fish 25 g (1 oz)

Shellfish 25 g (1 oz)

HIGH-PROTEIN FOODS
These high-protein foods, in these portions, all produce 6 g of protein.

Lean meat 25 g (1 oz)

Camembert 40 g (1½ oz)

Cheddar cheese 25 g (1 oz)

Nuts 25 g (1 oz) incomplete

Milk 190 ml (6½ fl oz)

Boiled rice 50 g (1¾ oz)

1 wholemeal biscuit

Boiled pasta 50 g (1¾ oz)

1 large slice bread

3 crackers

INCOMPLETE PROTEINS
These foods, in these amounts, all provide 2 g of incomplete protein, though not necessarily the same type.

Breakfast cereal 25 g (1 oz)

Corn on the cob 50 g (1¾ oz)

Oatmeal porridge 15 g (½ oz)

Potatoes 140 g (5 oz)

THE KIDNEYS AND EXCESS PROTEIN

As part of the urinary tract, the kidneys have two main functions: filtering the blood and excreting waste products and excess water. The most important waste products are those generated by the breakdown of proteins. Proteins have a high nitrogen content, which is dangerous to the body, and this must be filtered out. If too many high-protein foods are eaten, the kidneys must work much harder to remove the waste matter. The increased level of urine that is needed to excrete the nitrogen puts a strain on the kidneys and may lead to renal disorders or damage to the kidneys' filtering units, the glomeruli. If the glomeruli are damaged, blood and protein will be lost in the urine. Mild versions of this condition occur naturally with age, but severe cases may ultimately lead to the destruction of the kidneys.

EXCRETING URINE
Excess amino acids that are not needed by the body are converted to urea in the liver. Urea travels via the bloodstream to the kidneys and is removed in urine.

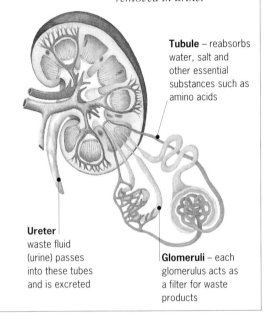

Tubule – reabsorbs water, salt and other essential substances such as amino acids

Ureter
waste fluid (urine) passes into these tubes and is excreted

Glomeruli – each glomerulus acts as a filter for waste products

Special needs
Broken bones and severe injury may cause significant loss of protein. A convalescent's diet should therefore be high in protein. If appetite is poor, offer fish, milk, eggs and nuts, which are often more appealing than meats, and prepare dishes supplemented with powdered milk, soya flour and dried yeast. Be sure, also, to provide adequate carbohydrates and fats to prevent the body using its supply of protein for energy.

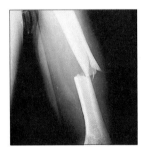

LOSING PROTEIN
About 60 grams of protein a day may be lost owing to injury.

such as a broken limb, need to increase significantly their protein intake to help the body repair the damage. Children's protein requirements are also greater than those of adults. They need it because their bodies are constantly laying down new tissue while they are growing. A month's deficiency may result in stunted growth and may even impair mental development.

Too little protein can upset the body's fluid balance. The body then retains water leading to oedema (fluid retention). The swollen stomachs of children in developing countries who suffer from kwashiorkor (protein malnutrition) are due to fluid retention.

DID YOU KNOW?
The essential amino acid phenylalanine forms part of the artificial sweetener aspartame, which is used in a wide range of sugar-free foods and beverages such as diet yoghurt and low-calorie colas. Although aspartame is considered a safe product by government health departments, it should always be used in moderation.

How much protein is too much?
While too little protein is certainly bad, many nutritionists believe that eating too much also may be harmful. The amount of protein you eat can easily build up. An excess of 200 grams of protein a day, which is more than four times what the body needs, can be consumed by eating a breakfast of pancakes and cream, a lunch of rice with chilli con carne and a glass of milk, a snack of peanuts, and a dinner that includes a baked potato topped with some grated cheese, with ice cream for dessert.

Such excessive amounts of protein place a strain on the kidneys. The body's tissues do not use the nitrogen part of the protein molecule and it is excreted by the kidneys. The more protein consumed, the more fluid the kidneys need to flush out the nitrogen.

Nor can the body store surplus protein. In the short term, protein is converted into glucose in the liver or directly combines with oxygen to provide heat and energy. Any protein that is not used in this way is converted to fat and stored. Therefore, in terms of food cost and the risk to health, eating too much protein is an expensive way for you to obtain energy. In addition,

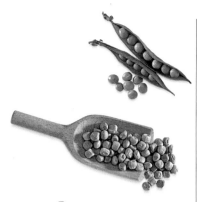

PODS AND PULSES
A green pea or a green bean with its pod is not termed a pulse. It is usually called a fresh vegetable. Pulses are the dried seeds of these pod-bearing plants. But, whether a pea or a bean is fresh, frozen or dried, it contains the same amount of protein.

animal protein, in the form of full-fat dairy products and fatty meat, is virtually always associated with high levels of saturated fat. So the more animal protein in your diet the more saturated fat you are likely to consume. In the long term, diets high in saturated fat have been linked to heart disease and stroke.

High protein (amino acid) supplements are often taken by athletes in the mistaken belief that this is the quickest way to make them stronger and more muscular. But consuming large amounts of protein does not help build more muscle: only exercise can build more muscle cells. Instead, athletes and others interested in body building in particular should eat more carbohydrate-rich foods, such as pasta, to provide them with the energy to carry out their intensive exercise programmes.

Studies have shown that eating too many protein-rich foods or taking purified amino acid supplements encourages the body to lose calcium in urine. Excess calcium loss causes osteoporosis (thinning of the bones), a serious condition that is on the rise among postmenopausal women (see p. 69). Those at risk should avoid high-protein foods, and make sure that they have sufficient intakes of calcium and vitamin D.

Pathway to health

Gout is a very painful disease that is caused by excess uric acid in the blood. This causes uric acid crystals to form in the joints, particularly the big toe. The joint becomes inflamed, swollen and very tender. The sufferer often experiences extreme pain and may be unable to put any pressure on the affected area. Usually, the first attack of gout affects only a single joint and may last for a few days. But if there are subsequent attacks, more joints may become affected.

Uric acid is made from the breakdown of nucleic acids (the material in the cell nucleus). Some protein foods, for example, kidneys and other offal, are high in nucleic acids. Some experts recommend that gout sufferers avoid these foods.

Naturopathy is commonly used to treat gout. Cherries are recommended by some practitioners for easing the pain. Sufferers from gout should also drink plenty of fluids and try to limit their intake of alcohol.

MEATLESS PROTEIN BOOSTS

If you want to restrict your meat intake but still retain protein in your diet, try these tasty meals and snacks. Combining a few nutritious foods will provide the right proportion of protein while adding variety to your diet.

▶ *Beans and grains – try tofu, lentils or beans served with rice; or felafel (deep-fried chickpea balls) in pitta bread. Because soya beans have a 41 to 50 per cent protein content, soya products such as soya milk, soya yoghurt and soya bean curd (tofu) have become popular with people who want to curtail their meat consumption.*

▶ *Use more beans and less meat in dishes such as chilli con carne. You will get plenty of protein while reducing the cost and fat content of the dish.*

▶ *Seeds or nuts and beans – the Middle Eastern dish, hummus (chickpea and sesame seed spread) or Chinese bean curd with sesame seeds are two popular combinations.*

▶ *Peanuts and grains – peanuts, which fall into the category of pulses, provide almost as much protein as beef when combined with grains. Spread peanut butter on wholemeal toast for a nourishing snack.*

MEXICAN DELIGHT
This hearty meal, which combines taco shells and beans, provides good-quality protein. Add some low-fat yoghurt and plenty of vegetables for a well-balanced meal.

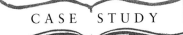

The Vegetarian Body Builder

For many people the major source of protein is meat, so vegetarians may well ask, 'How will I get enough protein?' For vegetarians who work out with weights, this question seems all the more pressing. After all, aren't body builders supposed to follow a protein-rich diet? What, therefore, are the foods these people need to eat?

Paul is 29 and single. Since his college days, he has been a vegetarian. Last year Paul noticed that he was gaining weight. His friend, Simon, suggested he join a gym and since then Paul has been lifting weights three times a week.

Although Paul made considerable progress in the first few months, his increase in stamina began to slow down. Simon suggested that the lack of protein in Paul's vegetarian diet was causing the problem.

Because Paul does not eat meat, he decided to try amino acid supplements, which are available from chemists and health food stores. After a few weeks he started to develop migraines, lost his appetite and had less energy. Now he is worried that something is wrong.

WHAT SHOULD PAUL DO?

Paul should make an appointment with his doctor to establish the cause of his symptoms. His doctor can also refer him to a dietitian. Analysing his diet will help Paul to find out whether he really does need to boost his protein intake with amino acid supplements.

Paul needs to consider whether weight training alone will help him to overcome his problem of excess weight. With his trainer, Paul could devise a new programme that will help him to further his gains in strength and stamina. He needs to investigate whether an aerobic exercise, such as swimming or cycling, will help to reduce his weight and keep it stable more effectively than just weight-training.

DIET
Lacking protein-rich meat in their diets, vegetarians need to make sure they are consuming the right combination of plant proteins.

HEALTH
Supplements can cause problems such as triggering migraines in susceptible people. It is wise to check with a doctor or nutritionist before taking them.

Action Plan

HEALTH
Consult doctor to find out what is the cause of the migraines, appetite loss and loss of energy.

DIET
Consult a dietitian to find out whether his diet contains sufficient protein. (The dietitian will teach Paul how to choose and combine vegetarian foods for a nutritionally well-balanced diet.)

FITNESS
Find out about other activities that will help to reduce weight and increase stamina. See whether the sports centre has aerobics classes.

HOW THINGS TURNED OUT FOR PAUL

Paul's doctor explained that the supplements contributed to his symptoms and would not aid muscle growth. His trainer suggested that on the days he did not work out, Paul could swim or cycle for at least half an hour to help lose surplus weight. Paul visited a dietitian who confirmed that his diet, which includes plenty of beans and wheat, is providing him with sufficient protein calories. After a few days without the supplements, Paul found the migraines had disappeared.

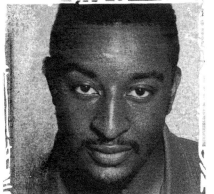

FITNESS
Following a single exercise programme may not be the best way of increasing stamina.

VEGETARIANISM

No longer viewed as just for eccentrics, a meatless diet is growing ever more popular, particularly with the young, as researchers discover the health benefits of meat-free eating.

WHAT IS A VEGETARIAN?

By definition, vegetarianism prohibits the consumption of meat or fish, but some diets are more restrictive than others.

▶ *Demi or semi-vegetarians eat fish, and sometimes chicken, but not red meat.*

▶ *Ovo-lacto-vegetarians include milk and eggs in their diet but not meat or fish.*

▶ *Lacto-vegetarians have milk and yoghurt, as well as cheese made with vegetarian rennet, but no meat, fish or eggs.*

▶ *Vegans do not eat any animal products at all, banning meat, fish, milk and eggs from their diets.*

▶ *Fruitarians exclude pulses and cereals from the diet as well as all foods of animal origin. Fruitarians eat only fruit, honey, nuts and nut oils.*

▶ *Macrobiotic followers have a diet consisting of ten different levels, which become progressively more restrictive. At first, animal foods are excluded, then fruit and vegetables as well. At the final 'purist' level only brown rice is eaten.*

In the United Kingdom, about 2.5 million people (4.3 per cent of the population) call themselves vegetarians. In the United States, the number of people making this claim is about 12.4 million (7 per cent of the population) and in Germany about 2.9 million people (4.5 per cent of the population) say they do not eat meat.

THE HEALTH BENEFITS

On the whole, vegetarians tend to follow current healthy eating guidelines. Because they do not eat meat, a prime source of saturated fat, vegetarians take in less total fat, as well as more fibre, in the form of fresh fruits, vegetables and wholegrain cereals. These foods are also good sources of beta carotene, vitamin C and vitamin E, which are antioxidant nutrients and may protect the body from disease (see p. 94).

The Oxford Vegetarian Study, a long-term project set up in 1980 by researchers at Oxford University, has collected information on the health and mortality of more than 6000 vegetarian subjects and a control group of more than 5000 meat-eating individuals. Allowing for smoking habits, body size and social class – all factors that influence mortality rates – the study has revealed significant differences between the two groups. For example, in contrast to meat eaters, vegetarians have a 39 per cent lower risk of dying from cancer.

The study's research team also found that the risk of heart disease was 24 per cent lower in vegetarians and 57 per cent lower in vegans than in regular meat eaters. And when their blood cholesterol concentrations were compared, researchers found vegetarians, particularly vegans, had lower levels of

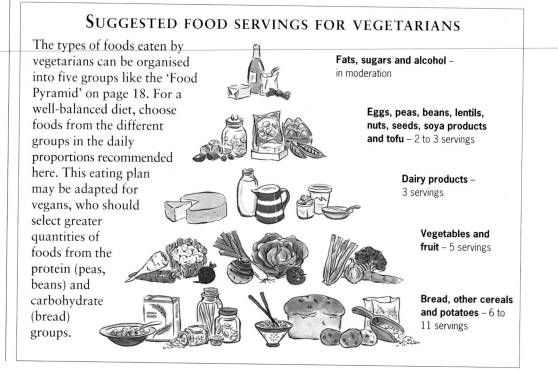

SUGGESTED FOOD SERVINGS FOR VEGETARIANS

The types of foods eaten by vegetarians can be organised into five groups like the 'Food Pyramid' on page 18. For a well-balanced diet, choose foods from the different groups in the daily proportions recommended here. This eating plan may be adapted for vegans, who should select greater quantities of foods from the protein (peas, beans) and carbohydrate (bread) groups.

Fats, sugars and alcohol – in moderation

Eggs, peas, beans, lentils, nuts, seeds, soya products and tofu – 2 to 3 servings

Dairy products – 3 servings

Vegetables and fruit – 5 servings

Bread, other cereals and potatoes – 6 to 11 servings

low-density lipoproteins (LDLs) – the 'bad' blood cholesterol, which is a primary risk factor in heart disease (see p. 56).

Another major study of 1900 vegetarians was conducted by researchers at the German Cancer Research Centre in 1978. The researchers found that the rate of cardiovascular disease was 61 per cent lower in male vegetarians and 44 per cent lower in female vegetarians than in the general population. The men in the study had a greatly reduced cancer death rate – about half the national average – and the women's cancer mortality rate was reduced by one quarter.

A vegetarian diet may also give some protection against colon cancer, and much research is being undertaken to determine why. Between 1980 and 1986 Walter C. Willett, a professor at Harvard Medical School, studied more than 88 000 women aged 34 to 59 years. His results showed that daily consumption of red meat more than doubled the risk of developing colon cancer, compared to eating such food less than once a week. But meat eaters usually eat fewer vegetables than vegetarians. It may be the lack of vegetables eaten rather than an excess of meat that was of significance in the study. Vegetables are a rich source of the antioxidants that may help to prevent cancer. The high fibre intake among vegetarians is considered to be another factor in lowering their risk of colon cancer.

Some researchers claim that premature death by cancer and heart disease is only part of the story for meat eaters. The high-protein diet that comes with eating meat may have other consequences. For example, calcium loss and increased uric acid from eating too much protein may be a cause of kidney stones, kidney failure and gout.

Eating a vegetarian diet may help to relieve the symptoms of rheumatoid arthritis, according to Dr Jens Kjeldsen-Kragh of the Institute of Immunology and Rheumatology at the National Hospital, Oslo, Norway. He found in 1991 that patients on an established vegetarian diet faced less pain and stiffness, and fewer swollen joints. However, sufferers of other types of arthritis such as ankylosing spondylitis, appear to benefit from a high-meat, low complex carbohydrate diet.

Citing these studies and many others, researchers now believe that vegetarianism may promote longevity. But their diet may

SOURCES OF PROTEIN IN A DAILY MENU

Many foods beside meat provide protein. The meals shown below contain a range of simple, nourishing foods that supply an adequate intake of protein.

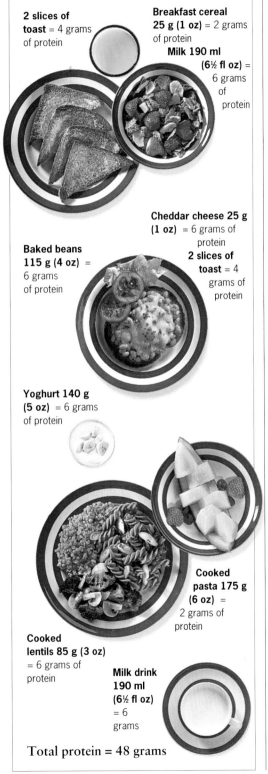

2 slices of toast = 4 grams of protein

Breakfast cereal 25 g (1 oz) = 2 grams of protein

Milk 190 ml (6½ fl oz) = 6 grams of protein

Cheddar cheese 25 g (1 oz) = 6 grams of protein

2 slices of toast = 4 grams of protein

Baked beans 115 g (4 oz) = 6 grams of protein

Yoghurt 140 g (5 oz) = 6 grams of protein

Cooked pasta 175 g (6 oz) = 2 grams of protein

Cooked lentils 85 g (3 oz) = 6 grams of protein

Milk drink 190 ml (6½ fl oz) = 6 grams

Total protein = 48 grams

Vegetarian cheese
Rennet, which is used in cheese-making, traditionally comes from the stomach lining of cows. Strict vegetarians often refuse to eat ordinary cheese because it contains this animal product. Luckily, cheeses are now available made with vegetarian rennet, which is genetically engineered from micro-organisms, and therefore does not require the rennet from animal sources.

Textured vegetable protein

An inexpensive alternative to meat, textured vegetable protein (TVP) is made from soya beans. First the oil is extracted and refined to make vegetable oil. Then the residue is processed to extract the protein, which is formed into a white spongy product that is available in an assortment of shapes and sizes. TVP is usually fortified with B vitamins and iron.

USING TEXTURED VEGETABLE PROTEIN
After soaking, TVP can be cooked in a variety of ways – try combining it with nuts and pulses in casseroles and roasts or use it to make vegetarian burgers.

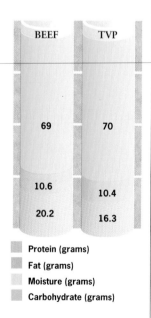

BEEF	TVP
69	70
10.6	10.4
20.2	16.3

- Protein (grams)
- Fat (grams)
- Moisture (grams)
- Carbohydrate (grams)

NUTRITIONAL VALUES
The bar chart above compares the nutritional content of beef and TVP.

not be the only reason why vegetarians are healthier than meat eaters. Vegetarians tend also to live 'healthier' lives – smoking and drinking alcohol less and exercising more.

Meeting your needs

With all these health benefits, it is little wonder that vegetarianism is becoming increasingly popular. But to be a healthy vegetarian, you need a balanced diet. It is not enough just to stop eating animal flesh and consume a few high-protein foods, such as cheese, instead. Cheese, like meat, contains a lot of fat, particularly saturated fat, which is linked to heart disease and cancer. Choose low-fat dairy products such as skimmed milk or low-fat yoghurt, and make sure that your diet includes foods from all the main vegetarian food groups: fresh fruit and vegetables; nuts, seeds, pulses and soya products; grains and cereals; and low-fat dairy products. With a little planning, you can make nourishing meals using a variety of fresh foods.

Missing nutrients?

Some people believe that a vegetarian diet does not offer an adequate supply of vitamins and minerals. But by eating a variety of foods vegetarians should get all the nutrients they need. They do have an increased risk of iron and zinc deficiency, however, especially if they eat large amounts of unleavened bread, for example, chapattis. These foods contain phytic acid, which inhibits mineral absorption.

Vegans may not get enough vitamin B_{12} and vitamin D. A prolonged deficiency of vitamin B_{12} may seriously impair the body's central nervous system, causing numbness in the limbs. In addition, there may be neurological signs such as loss of memory.

A good supply of vitamin D is also essential for the healthy development of bones in infants and children. Many foods are fortified with these vitamins. Vitamin B_{12} is added during processing to some vegetarian burgers, as well as to breakfast cereals, yeast extract and soya milk. Most margarines are fortified with vitamin D. Adults who receive sufficient sunlight can synthesise adequate amounts of vitamin D from cholesterol in the skin. Just 15 minutes of exposure to sunlight per day is sufficient for most adults. However, some vegetarians, especially those on a macrobiotic diet, may require supplements for optimum health; so if you are in any doubt you should consult your doctor.

A VEGETARIAN IN THE FAMILY

Preparing and cooking meals for a vegetarian is easy even if everybody else eats meat. And meat eaters in the family may be persuaded to become 'part-time vegetarians' if the family has one or two meat-free days a week.

While many meals can be prepared without using any animal products, it is also possible to organise your meals so that you cater for both meat eaters and vegetarians with essentially the same dish. Instead of cooking two different meals, prepare a meat-free sauce, rice dish or casserole then divide it. Add beans and vegetables to one portion and meat or fish to the other.

SATISFYING DIFFERENT TASTES
Baked potatoes make a hearty meal and can be dressed with a variety of simple, nutritious toppings suitable for both vegetarians and meat eaters.

When making meat-free stews or soups, cook twice as much as you need and freeze the remainder in meal-size portions. These can be defrosted when you need a substitute for a meat dish for one member of the family. Leftover vegetable or textured vegetable protein mixtures can be used as alternative fillings for pies, sweet peppers or pancakes traditionally filled with meat.

For a meat eater, just add minced lean beef or chopped poultry to the vegetarian sauce

For a vegetarian, try beans lightly cooked with tomatoes, herbs and sweet peppers

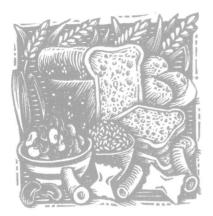

CHAPTER 3

THE OPTIMUM BODY FUEL – CARBOHYDRATES

Until recently, complex carbohydrates, in the form of starchy foods such as bread, potatoes, pasta, rice and cereals, were generally frowned upon by nutritionists because their starch content was held to be a major cause of obesity. Many sugary foods are still considered to be unhealthy because of their high fat content, and so harmful to health, but carbohydrates in their more complex form are now seen as satisfying rather than fattening and are an essential source of energy.

THE ENERGY FOODS

Although starchy and sweet foods look and taste different, they are all primarily made up of the same building block – sugar – the body's best source of energy.

Polysaccharide

Monosaccharide

Disaccharide

SUGAR UNITS
All carbohydrates are made up of molecules called saccharides. Simple sugars, such as glucose and fructose, consist of single ring-like units (monosaccharides). Table sugar (sucrose) is a disaccharide that is made up of two monosaccharides, glucose and fructose, connected by an oxygen molecule. Complex carbohydrates, or polysaccharides, are long, spiralling chains of many connecting monosaccharides that are usually glucose.

Whenever you lift a weight, go for a walk or run for a bus, your body relies on its various sources of energy to keep you going. The body's primary source of energy is carbohydrate, a group of foods with similar chemical components that is divided into two categories: simple sugars and complex carbohydrates.

The simplest of sugars consist of single molecules called monosaccharides and include glucose, fructose and galactose. Glucose occurs naturally only in fruits and honey and is the only carbohydrate used directly by the body to generate energy.

Disaccharides, which form when two molecules join up include sucrose (table sugar), lactose (milk sugar) and maltose (malt sugar). Complex carbohydrates, also known as starches, are made up of at least ten saccharides and are found in many plant foods like wheat, rice, potatoes, cornmeal, yams and green bananas.

Most carbohydrates are broken down into glucose when digested; the rest are changed to glucose in the liver. If the body does not need carbohydrates for energy immediately, the muscles and liver store them as glycogen, which then provides

IS SUGAR BAD FOR HEALTH?

Sugar has been accused of contributing to many diseases and disorders, including diabetes, heart disease, hypertension, and hyperactivity in children. But research studies have not provided evidence that sugar actually causes any of these conditions. What most nutritionists will confirm, however, is that the frequent consumption of sugar accelerates tooth decay.

Everybody has bacteria in the mouth that can form plaque (a film of mucus) on teeth. Sugar or starch that remains in the mouth becomes easily accessible food for the bacteria, which produce an acid that damages tooth enamel and causes cavities. Tooth decay is most strongly linked to the frequency of sugar consumption and the propensity for the sweet foods to cling to the teeth. Toffees, hard sweets and chewing gum, therefore, are more cariogenic than cakes.

It is better if sweet foods or sugary drinks are consumed with meals rather than between meals.

The role of sugar in obesity is more complex, since it is the total number of calories consumed that is important, rather than the calorie source. However, many sugary foods such as ice cream, cakes, biscuits and chocolates are also high in fat; people who eat large amounts of them may find that cutting down on these foods aids weight loss.

DENTAL FLOSSING
Acid only forms on teeth if plaque is present. It is important to clean and floss your teeth regularly to remove plaque.

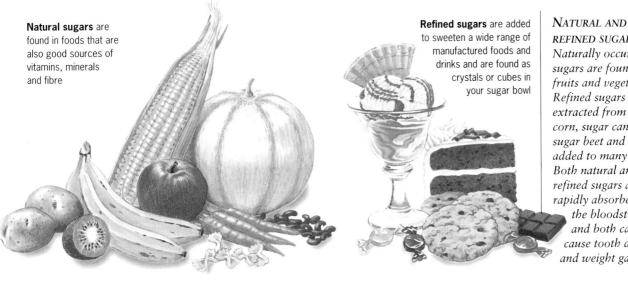

Natural sugars are found in foods that are also good sources of vitamins, minerals and fibre

Refined sugars are added to sweeten a wide range of manufactured foods and drinks and are found as crystals or cubes in your sugar bowl

NATURAL AND REFINED SUGARS Naturally occurring sugars are found in fruits and vegetables. Refined sugars are extracted from fruit, corn, sugar cane or sugar beet and are added to many foods. Both natural and refined sugars are rapidly absorbed into the bloodstream and both can cause tooth decay and weight gain.

THE CARBOHYDRATE CONTENT OF FOOD

Many foods contain both simple sugars and complex carbohydrates, and the relative proportions of these are shown in the table below. Foods at the top of the table are high in sugars, while those at the bottom are high in starches. Think of the table as a traffic light, with 'red' at the top, 'amber' in the centre and 'green for go' foods at the bottom. Ideally, eat no more than 55 grams (2 ounces) of added sugar a day (see p. 42), preferably in high-fibre desserts, cakes and biscuits such as oatmeal biscuits or banana bread.

FOOD	COMPLEX CARBOHYDRATES grams per portion	SUGARS grams per portion	COMMENTS
'RED FOODS'			
Boiled sweets, 10 average	0.3	60.8	Almost pure sugar.
Sweetened puffed wheat cereal, 40 g (1½ oz)	11.2	22.6	High in added sugar and low in fibre.
Sponge cake, 1 slice, 55 g (2 oz)	13.2	18	Cakes are high in added sugar.
Peaches canned in syrup, 115 g (4 oz)	0	16	At least half the sugar is added to fruit canned in syrup.
'AMBER FOODS'			
Fruit yoghurt, 115 g (4 oz)	0	20.5	Unflavoured yoghurt with fresh fruit is preferable.
Banana, 1 medium-size	3.0	31.4	Sugars in fruit and vegetables are encouraged.
Baked beans, 135 g (4¾ oz)	20.7	8	Added sugar makes beans palatable, particularly for children.
'GREEN FOODS'			
Sweet corn kernels, 25 g (1 oz)	5.0	2.9	Good sources of complex carbohydrates. These foods also provide other important nutrients. Protein is found in pasta and bread, magnesium in brown rice, potassium in potatoes, phosphorus in corn, and several B vitamins in bread. All unrefined, complex-carbohydrate foods are good sources of dietary fibre.
Jacket potato, 140 g (5 oz)	44	1.7	
Rice, brown, 140 g (5 oz), cooked	47.4	1.1	
Rice, white, 140 g (5 oz), cooked	44.4	0	
Bread, wholegrain, 1 slice, 25 g (1 oz)	11.9	0.5	
Pasta, white, 225 g (8 oz), cooked	50	0.7	
Bread, white, 1 slice, 25 g (1 oz)	14	0.8	

41

Sweeteners

Manufacturers add sugar as a sweetener to many different processed foods. But it is not always easy to know that they have done so, since it is listed on the label under many different names. For example, corn syrup, dextrose, maltose, maltodextrin, glucose syrup, invert sugar and levulose are all forms of sugar.

SPICED DELIGHT
Use sweet flavourings such as cinnamon, allspice, cardamom, cloves, ginger and nutmeg when you prepare foods and reduce your sugar intake without reducing flavour.

energy when the body demands it. Any surplus glucose is eventually converted to fat and stored in the body.

Extra goodness

Unrefined carbohydrates, such as breads, wholegrain cereals and brown rice, are highly nutritious. But, when they are refined as white sugar and white flour, carbohydrates lose much of their nutritional value. Unrefined foods are particularly good for you because they are usually full of fibre. Dietary fibre plays a major role in bowel function (see p. 46). Research suggests that insoluble fibre may help to prevent bowel cancers and soluble fibre may help to lower the blood cholesterol level. In addition, complex carbohydrate foods, such as dried beans and root vegetables, provide not only starch and fibre but also essential vitamins and minerals.

A CHANGE FOR THE WORSE

In affluent societies, the most dramatic dietary change in the past 100 years has been the switch from complex carbohydrate foods to foods that are high in fat and sugar. These high-fat and refined-sugar diets are generally low in fibre. The combination of these factors is thought to contribute to several contemporary disease concerns – particularly tooth decay, heart disease, cancer and bowel disorders – that have arisen over the same period. Most health experts recommend returning to a diet more like that of agricultural societies – with more complex carbohydrate foods and less sugar and fat.

Added sugar: sweet poison

Manufacturers often add refined sugar to food because it has important preservative properties; it also adds bulk and viscosity to foods. Fruit yoghurts, for example may contain the equivalent of five teaspoons of sugar. Sweetening natural low-fat yoghurt with your own fresh fruit, such as blackberries, apricots or strawberries is a much healthier alternative.

Unlike foods rich in complex carbohydrates, those high in refined sugars are often poor sources of other nutrients; for this reason, they are often called 'empty calories'. Foods such as cakes, biscuits, doughnuts, sweets and chocolate are high in refined sugar and do not have any compensating nutrients or fibre.

Certain foods, such as baked beans and a few high-fibre breakfast cereals contain added simple sugars to make them tastier. However, since these foods are a good source of other important nutrients and the amount of sugar is not excessive, they can still be a valuable part of a healthy diet. It is worth consuming sugar with foods that provide other nutrients. Even though they contain sugars, fruit and milk (especially reduced-fat milk) are good for you and should be part of a healthy diet because they offer vitamins, minerals and, in the case of milk, protein.

MORE THAN JUST DAILY BREAD

There are a number of ways that you can add more complex carbohydrate foods to your diet while cutting down on fatty and sugary foods. All types of bread are good

SATISFYING YOUR SWEET TOOTH

From birth, babies seem to prefer sweet to sour tastes. Most adults and almost all children enjoy sweet-tasting foods. But cutting back on sugar does not mean denying yourself sweet foods or desserts. Fruits contain natural sugars so by using unsweetened fruit juice, fresh fruit and unsweetened canned fruit to replace refined sugars in recipes, you satisfy your sweet tooth without harming your health. The benefits are obvious – less tooth decay, and more vitamins and fibre.

Here are some suggestions:

► *If fresh fruit is not available, eat fruits canned in unsweetened fruit juice rather than syrup.*

► *Substitute fresh fruit purées for sugar in recipes, if possible.*

► *Add fresh fruit to natural yoghurt.*

► *Sprinkle sweet spices on foods, for example, cinnamon with baked apples.*

► *Choose processed foods in which the sugar has been replaced partially by an artificial sweetener, such as aspartame or acesulfame K.*

for you, so eat more bread. Although white bread is fortified with vitamins and minerals, replacing nutrients that are lost when flour is refined, wholemeal bread provides more fibre. Thicker slices mean that you get more bread in proportion to the amount of butter or jam – a good way to cut down on the total calories eaten.

Starting the day with cereal will help to provide you with a steady stream of energy during the morning. Porridge and other wholegrain breakfast cereals are full of nutrients as well as complex carbohydrates. By using reduced-fat milk, you can make sure that you do not take in unneeded fat. Then choose snacks that are rich in carbohydrates and low in fat. Wholewheat biscuits, breadsticks and pitta bread filled with salad are both tasty and good for you.

Dried beans provide both starch and fibre. When making meat dishes, replace one-third of the meat with dried beans. Also add beans to salads, soups and stews, and purée them to make spreads and dips.

Base desserts on fruit and cereals: make a fruit salad instead of a fruit pie, try frozen natural low-fat yoghurt with a toasted oatmeal topping, and sweeten rice pudding with fresh or dried fruit.

LOSING WEIGHT

Since foods high in complex carbohydrates are filling, chewy, and full of fibre and other nutrients, they are ideal for people who want to lose weight. Because the majority of calories in many people's diets came from carbohydrates, dieters used to have the mistaken idea that carbohydrate foods are fattening. Some diet books also wrongly claimed that overweight people had a defective capacity for dealing with carbohydrates and that these foods led to deposits of fat.

DOES YOUR CARBOHYDRATE INTAKE MEASURE UP?

The current recommendations for healthy eating suggest that you should obtain about 50 to 60 per cent of your energy needs (calories) from complex carbohydrates. Most nutritionists agree that consumption of refined sugars should be reduced to about 10 per cent of your calorie intake.

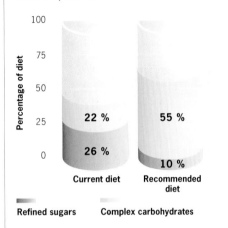

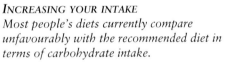

INCREASING YOUR INTAKE
Most people's diets currently compare unfavourably with the recommended diet in terms of carbohydrate intake.

Moral crusade
During the 19th century, a crusade against refined wheat flour was led by the Reverend Sylvester Graham (1794–1851). A Presbyterian minister from Philadelphia, Graham fiercely condemned white bread, claiming it was contributing to the downfall of society.

Graham described the refining process as putting 'asunder what God has joined together'. He encouraged people to eat more wholegrain bread and wrote a long treatise on its importance for the moral, spiritual and physical welfare of mankind. Subsequently, wholewheat flour was named after him, and all Americans are familiar with the 'Graham cracker' – a healthy, wholewheat biscuit.

PUTTING HEALTH ON YOUR PLATE

Most people should eat plenty of complex carbohydrate foods. One of the easiest ways to do this is to rethink the proportions of food you put on your plate. Rice, pasta, bread and potatoes should fill two-fifths of the plate, vegetables or salad should make up at least another two-fifths, and meat, fish, cheese or eggs the remainder.

IN THE RIGHT PROPORTION
Savoury rice and a crisp green salad make up four-fifths of this well-balanced meal planned with the food pyramid (see p. 18) in mind. A small piece of salmon supplies the protein.

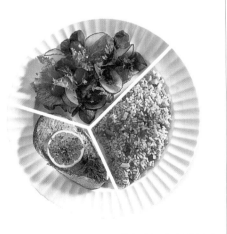

Plain is best

Gram for gram, ounce for ounce, fatty foods are more than twice as high in calories as complex carbohydrates. But while starchy foods such as pasta and potatoes are naturally low in calories, adding butter or an oily dressing negates this benefit.

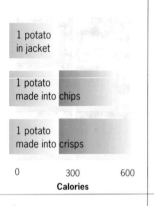

1 potato
in jacket

1 potato
made into chips

1 potato
made into crisps

0   300   600
Calories

ACCUMULATING CALORIES
An average baked potato provides about 200 calories. Once peeled and fried, the same potato offers about 500 calories; if made into potato crisps, the potato would then be valued at 600 calories.

Nutritionists now know that it is the total calorie content of the diet, along with the amount of exercise taken, that determines whether a person is likely to lose, maintain or gain weight, and that fat is often the culprit in overweight or obesity.

Reducing your fat intake is one of the most effective ways of reducing your total calorie intake, because one gram of fat has nine calories while one gram of carbohydrate or protein has only four calories.

Proteins versus carbohydrates

Dieters were once encouraged to make their meals high in protein rather than carbohydrates, and many people still believe that weight loss will be more successful on high-protein, low-carbohydrate diets. However, high-protein foods, such as meat and cheese, are often high in fat and are therefore not low in calories. Diets high in protein and low in carbohydrate are also likely to be low in fibre, which makes them less

Pathway to health

If you are very concerned about being overweight, talk to your doctor and ask him or her for a referral to a dietitian. The dietitian will recommend a weight-loss diet that best suits your needs and personality and will also monitor your progress.

satisfying, resulting in the craving for larger amounts. Most experts argue that weight loss is most easily achieved by cutting down on the intake of fat without altering the intake of carbohydrates. For a diet to be successful, however, dieters must be careful not to cook or dress the carbohydrate foods with oil and fat.

Large quantities of low-fat, high-bulk foods are actually likely to help you lose weight. In one experiment, a group of young Irishmen were put on a diet that involved eating just under one kilogram (about two pounds) of potatoes a day for three months. Provided that they ate the potatoes, they were allowed to eat as much other food as they wanted. However, after three months most of the men had lost weight. They found that by filling themselves up with the potatoes they automatically reduced their total intake of other high-calorie foods.

Most health experts agree that it is not easy to lose weight. Keeping to a strict dietary regime for a few weeks often results in the loss of a few pounds, but it is very difficult to stick to it for long, and the pounds soon creep back when dietary habits return to normal. Therefore, changing the balance of your diet over the long term to one that is high in complex carbohydrate foods and lower in foods with a high-fat content is a more successful method of maintaining weight loss.

'HEAVEN'S GIFT'

Honey is a smooth, sticky sweetener, which the Roman poet Virgil called 'heaven's gift'. It has been enjoyed by humans for thousands of years.

The simple sugars, glucose and fructose, which give honey its sweetness, tasting even sweeter than table sugar (sucrose, also a simple sugar). This is where honey's real value lies. Less of it is needed to sweeten food than sugar and, because honey has a high-water content, it contains fewer calories than sugar for the same amount in weight. There are 385 calories in 100 grams (3½ ounces) of sugar, while only 304 calories in 100 grams (3½ ounces) of honey. But honey is still a sugar food, so limit its use.

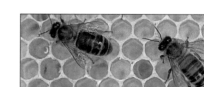
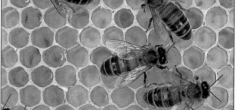

HONEY FACTORY
Worker honeybees fill the honeycomb, a waxy cylindrical network, with nectar from flowers. The chambers are capped with wax, and the honey is left to ripen for a few weeks.

HIGH-FIBRE SATISFACTION

Compare the types and amounts of food in the two sample meals shown below. Both have similar calorie counts and both provide protein, vitamins and minerals. But the meal high in fibre has more bulk and is far more satisfying.

MENU ONE
Meals high in fibre.

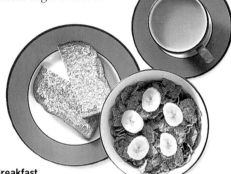

Breakfast
25 g (1 oz) wholewheat flakes
with semi-skimmed milk and 1 small sliced banana;
1 slice wholemeal bread or toast with 1 tsp butter or margarine; coffee with semi-skimmed milk = 5.3 g of fibre

Mid morning
Coffee with 30 ml (2 tbsp) semi-skimmed milk = 0 g of fibre

Lunch
2 wholemeal rolls with 1 tsp mayonnaise, filled with 115 g (4 oz) tuna and plain yoghurt, and a small salad; 225 ml (8 fl oz) semi-skimmed milk, apple and 140 g (5 oz) plain yoghurt = 7.4 g of fibre

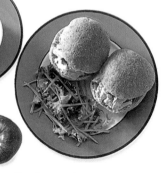

Evening meal
85 g (3 oz) chicken (cut in strips) stir-fried with broccoli, red pepper, spring onion; 115 g (4 oz) brown rice; 115 g (4 oz) fruit salad = 6.1 g of fibre

Bedtime
225 ml (8 fl oz) semi-skimmed milk = 0 g of fibre

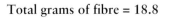

Total grams of fibre = 18.8

MENU TWO
Meals low in fibre.

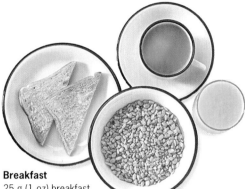

Breakfast
25 g (1 oz) breakfast cereal with semi-skimmed milk; 1 slice white toast with 1 tsp butter or margarine; 125 ml (4 fl oz) fruit juice (orange); coffee with semi-skimmed milk = 0.8 g of fibre

Mid morning
Coffee with 30 ml (2 tbsp) semi-skimmed milk = 0 g of fibre

Lunch
1 white roll with 1 tsp mayonnaise, filled with 25 g (1 oz) Cheddar cheese and salad; 225 ml (8 fl oz) semi-skimmed milk, banana and fruit-flavoured yoghurt =2.5 g of fibre

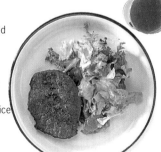

Evening meal
225 g (8 oz) grilled rump steak; 100 g (3½ oz) green salad with 1 tbsp vinaigrette dressing; 225 ml (8 fl oz) tomato juice = 4.6 g of fibre

Bedtime
225 ml (8 fl oz) semi-skimmed milk = 0 g of fibre

Total grams of fibre = 7.9

Artificial sugars
If you want to reduce your intake of table sugar (sucrose), you can add non-caloric, artificial sugars, such as aspartame and saccharin, to drinks and cold foods instead. They are also used by manufacturers to sweeten diet drinks like colas.

Saccharin has been available for over 50 years and is generally considered to be safe. Although studies on laboratory rats have shown that large quantities can cause bladder cancer, there have been no reports of it causing cancer in humans.

Aspartame is made up of two amino acids – aspartic acid and phenylalanine. After digestion, the amino acids are absorbed and used by the body like other amino acids (see p. 30).

Both saccharin and aspartame are 150 times sweeter than sugar, but they do not cause tooth decay. It is unwise to consume large amounts of artificial sweeteners, however, since the long-term effects of high intakes in humans is still unknown.

THE FIBRE FACTOR

During the 1980s, fibre was hailed as a way to halt colon cancer and to lower blood cholesterol. But despite this, many people have only slightly increased their fibre intake.

Oat bran

As a rich source of soluble fibre, oat bran is a valuable ally in the battle against excessive levels of harmful forms of cholesterol. In the 1980s medical reports trumpeting its particular benefits brought about an increase in its consumption. In fact, other foods that are high in soluble fibre – such as beans, apples, rolled oats and potatoes – are just as valuable as oat bran for reducing blood cholesterol.

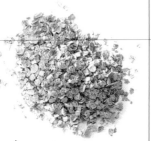

A VALUABLE INGREDIENT

On a cold day, a hot oat cereal makes a warming breakfast. Adding oats to desserts such as pancakes or apple crumble is another way to boost the nutritional value with extra fibre.

Although the role that fibre plays in stimulating bowel function has been well known since ancient times, its significance for disease prevention is a more recent discovery. Two British doctors, Denis Burkitt and Hugh Trowell, are credited with bringing this to the attention of the public in the 1970s. Having worked extensively in East Africa, they put forward the theory that many diseases common in industrialised countries but rare in Africa might be partly due to insufficient fibre in the Western diet. Further studies led to a consensus that people in the West could benefit from increasing the level of fibre content in their diets.

INSOLUBLE AND SOLUBLE FIBRE

The word *fibre* refers to a range of plant materials – components of plant cell walls – that the human body cannot digest. Other terms that are used to describe dietary fibre are *roughage* or *non-starch polysaccharides* (NSP). Most fibre compounds pass through the body unchanged until they reach the large intestine. Here, fibres act in different ways, depending on whether they are insoluble or soluble.

Insoluble fibre absorbs water, thus adding bulk to faecal matter in the bowel. This added bulk helps to stimulate the muscles of the lower digestive tract to move waste products more quickly. More importantly, insoluble fibre is fermented by bacteria in the large bowel to produce fatty acids that nourish the intestinal wall.

Diets that are low in insoluble fibre are associated with the need to 'strain' when passing a stool. Insufficient insoluble fibre is thought to contribute to such health problems as constipation, haemorrhoids and diverticulosis (protruding pockets formed on the intestinal wall that are prone to infection). By speeding waste material

INSOLUBLE AND SOLUBLE FIBRE IN FOODS

Wheat, rice, bran, wholegrain cereals and breads, and nuts are valuable sources of insoluble fibre. Soluble fibre foods include oats, oat bran, peas, beans, root vegetables and citrus fruits. Both types of fibre are found in apples, pears, barley, bananas, prunes and cabbages.

HIGH-FIBRE FOODS

The foods illustrated in the left circle provide insoluble fibre. The foods in the circle on the right are good sources of soluble fibre. In the middle are foods that provide both types of fibre.

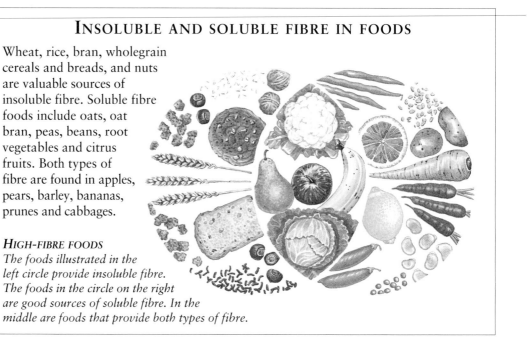

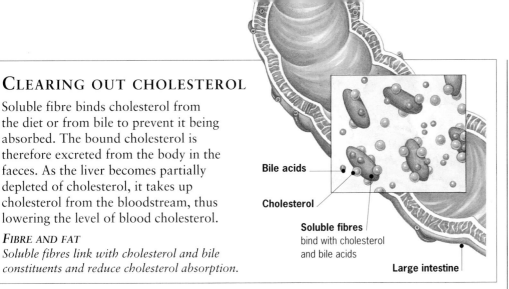

CLEARING OUT CHOLESTEROL

Soluble fibre binds cholesterol from the diet or from bile to prevent it being absorbed. The bound cholesterol is therefore excreted from the body in the faeces. As the liver becomes partially depleted of cholesterol, it takes up cholesterol from the bloodstream, thus lowering the level of blood cholesterol.

FIBRE AND FAT
Soluble fibres link with cholesterol and bile constituents and reduce cholesterol absorption.

Bile acids

Cholesterol

Soluble fibres
bind with cholesterol and bile acids

Large intestine

Slowly does it
Introduce high-fibre foods gradually into your diet to give your body time to adjust. You will also need to drink more, since fibre absorbs water. Because certain high-fibre foods – including dried peas, beans and lentils – often lead to increased flatulence, you may want to start by eating more cereals, grains, vegetables and fruits and then add pulses later.

through the body and therefore helping to prevent toxins from coming into prolonged contact with the intestinal wall, insoluble fibre may also protect against cancer of the lower bowel.

Soluble fibre compounds, as the term suggests, break down somewhat in the digestive tract and form fatty acids, which are absorbed into the bloodstream. These fatty acids are thought to help reduce the level of cholesterol in the blood, and therefore the risk of heart and arterial disease. In one study of men with high cholesterol levels, adding half a cup of cooked dried beans per day to their normal food intake reduced blood cholesterol levels by 13 per cent in 21 days.

Soluble fibre is also thought to delay the absorption of glucose into the bloodstream, helping to prevent diabetes mellitus and high blood sugar levels (hyperglycaemia).

HIGH FIBRE AND WEIGHT LOSS

Foods that are high in fibre are generally filling and low in fat and so can help to reduce total calorie intake. The chewiness of high-fibre foods prolongs eating time. Eating more slowly in turn gives your body time to tell your brain that your stomach is full. Another advantage is that larger portions of high-fibre foods often give you a similar calorie intake to smaller portions of refined foods. For example, 25 grams (1 ounce) of milk chocolate provide a similar calorie value (about 140 calories) as a medium-size (115 gram/4 ounce) baked potato eaten with its skin.

Since there are several ways of measuring the fibre content of foods, recommendations about how much fibre to eat vary. Generally speaking, 18 grams of fibre is a reasonable goal – a third as much again as adults in the developed world typically eat.

INCREASING THE FIBRE IN YOUR DIET

Nutritionists recommend that everybody should eat 18 grams of fibre a day to help digestion, lower cholesterol and prevent cancer of the bowel. Because people tend to eat too many refined foods, they miss out on the fibre they would get from unrefined products. An easy way to increase your intake of fibre is to include a variety of the foods listed right in your daily diet. The 'Food Pyramid' on page 18 will show you how to achieve the right balance.

CEREALS AND GRAINS
Wholegrain breakfast cereal (50 g/1¼ oz) = 6.5 g fibre
Wholemeal spaghetti, boiled (100 g/3½ oz) = 3.5 g fibre
Wholemeal bread (2 slices) = 3 g fibre

VEGETABLES AND FRUIT
Dried apricots (100 g/3½ oz) = 6.3 g fibre
Potato in skin (200 g/7 oz) = 5.4 g fibre
Apple with skin (140 g/5 oz) = 2.7 g fibre
Carrots (100 g/3½ oz) = 2.5 g fibre
Green beans (85 g/3 oz) = 2 g fibre
Raspberries (85 g/3 oz) = 2 g fibre

PEAS, BEANS AND LENTILS
Red kidney beans, or butter beans (100 g/3½ oz) = 4 g fibre
Lentils, cooked (200 g/7 oz) = 4 g fibre

YOUR DAILY INTAKE
Include some of these items in your diet to help increase your intake to 18 grams.

SUSTAINING ENERGY

Throughout the day, your energy level rises and falls as the sugars from the carbohydrates you eat enter your bloodstream and are used to provide energy.

Simple sugars are rapidly absorbed into the bloodstream after consumption, resulting in a sudden increase in blood sugar (glucose) concentration. Although the body breaks down starches to simple sugars, digestion and conversion must occur before absorption; therefore these sugars reach the bloodstream more slowly.

BLOOD SUGAR LEVELS

Most healthy people can tolerate sudden surges in blood sugar (glucose) concentration. But diabetics, who are deficient in insulin, are unable readily to control high blood sugar levels. Individuals who have been diabetic since childhood require extra insulin to control blood sugar levels, but many people who develop diabetes in middle age (adult-onset diabetes) can often control their blood sugar levels by adhering to a diet that is rich in complex carbohydrates and fibre, particularly soluble fibre. Soluble fibre helps to ensure that glucose is absorbed from the intestine into the bloodstream at a steady rate (see p. 47).

The brain and nervous system are sensitive to blood sugar concentrations. High blood sugar makes you feel sleepy; a low concentration makes you feel dizzy. Most people adapt to changes in blood sugar levels without experiencing serious symptoms, but there are some individuals who may experience symptoms of glucose deprivation, or hypoglycaemia, if their blood sugar levels fall rapidly. Hypoglycaemia is characterised by anxiety, dizziness, hunger, rapid heartbeat and weakness.

These effects can be countered quickly with a nourishing snack. People who suffer from hypoglycaemia need to eat a balanced diet and to eat regularly during the day. They should have high-fibre, complex carbohydrate snacks, such as a piece of fresh fruit, raw vegetables or slice of wholemeal bread, between meals.

This type of hypoglycaemia should not be confused with the low blood sugar levels which are associated with diabetes. If you are worried, consult your doctor, who will be able to make the correct diagnosis.

EATING TO BEST EFFECT Studies have shown that diabetics benefit greatly from eating a complex carbohydrate/high-fibre diet. Sufferers eating a low-fibre diet, especially if sugary foods are included, tend to have rapid increases in blood sugar levels. But foods such as beans, cereals and vegetables create a slow, steady rise in blood sugar levels. This allows sufferers to control their diabetes more effectively.

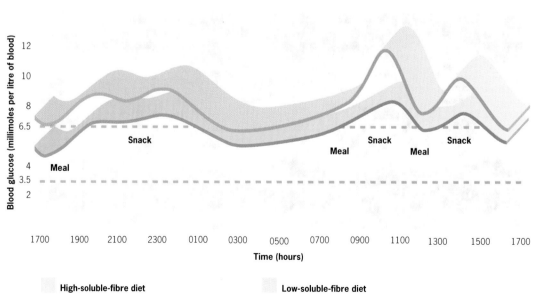

High-soluble-fibre diet   Low-soluble-fibre diet

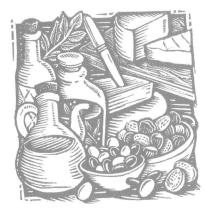

CHAPTER 4

THE IMPORTANCE OF FATS

*High consumption of foods containing
a lot of saturated fat was first linked to heart
disease less than 30 years ago. Since then, many
people have changed their eating habits – throwing
out their deep-fat fryers and buying leaner cuts of
meats. But some fats, especially the unsaturated fat
in certain oils, are vital to a healthy diet. Fats are an
excellent source of energy. They facilitate the
absorption of fat-soluble vitamins, and certain
fatty acids are essential for good health.*

A VITAL NUTRIENT

To be sure that your diet is healthy, you need to know which types of fats and oils are good for you, and which are harmful, as well as how much you need.

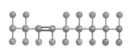

Saturated fatty acid

Monounsaturated fatty acid

Polyunsaturated fatty acid

● **Hydrogen** atoms
● **Carbon** atoms

SATURATION LEVELS
The number of hydrogen atoms a fatty acid chain holds determines its level of saturation. A saturated fatty acid chain carries a full set of these hydrogen atoms, which makes it harder to break up in the body. Saturated fats are major culprits in heart disease. In monounsaturated fats, only one pair of atoms is missing, while in polyunsaturated fats, two or more pairs are missing. These fats help to decrease the risk of heart disease.

Not all types of fat are created alike or equal; some are responsible for clogging the arteries and contribute to heart disease and stroke, others decrease the risk of thickened and blocked arteries.

At one time, people commonly breakfasted on bacon, eggs and buttered toast and drank their coffee with full-cream milk, then ate a lunch consisting of a cheese sandwich and a piece of fruit pie with custard. Dinner consisted of meat, at least two vegetables and another dessert. Vegetables were covered in butter, potatoes were fried, and very often the meat was beef, preferably well-marbled and served with a gravy made from the pan juices.

Today this diet reads like a recipe for a heart attack as all of these foods contain fat, and fatty foods have become the forbidden fruits of modern eating. The reason

that fat has become unpopular is that study after study has shown that the more of certain kinds of fat people eat, the more likely they are to develop heart disease. Although as yet controversial, evidence also seems to show a link between a fatty diet and some cancers, particularly those of the breast, bowel and pancreas. Since heart disease and cancer are the leading causes of death for adults in the developed world, excess dietary fat is considered a major health hazard. But this is not to say that all fats are bad for you. In fact, a diet that contains no fat can be just as dangerous as one that contains too much.

The human body could not function without fat. Every cell in the body contains fatty substances in its membranes. Fats also help the body to produce many hormones, some of which are related to fertility, while

FATS IN FOODS

A wide range of foods contains fat, and almost all foods contain more than one single type. Highest in saturated fats are meat and dairy products. The fattiest parts are the streaks or layers of visible fat on meat and the skin of chickens and other poultry. Processed foods, such as crisps, biscuits and ready-made meals, as

well as cakes, doughnuts and pies usually contain large amounts of fat, much of which is saturated.

Polyunsaturated and monounsaturated fats are found in fish, nuts and seeds. Even olive oil, which is mainly monounsaturated fat, contains 14 per cent saturated fat (see chart on page 52).

SATURATED FAT
Poultry skin, well-marbled meat, egg yolk, cheese and many processed foods are high in saturated fat.

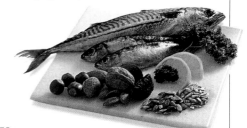

UNSATURATED FATS
Mackerel, sardines, nuts and seeds provide polyunsaturated fat. Olive and rapeseed oils are high in monounsaturated fat.

IS BUTTER BETTER THAN MARGARINE?

For years experts said that unsaturated fats, such as corn oil, were healthier than saturated fats, such as butter. Based on this advice, many people switched from butter to margarine believing that it was a healthier alternative. But new evidence shows that when liquid vegetable oils are made into solid margarine by the chemical process called hydrogenation, some of the fats in the oil are changed into substances called trans-fatty acids. The body metabolises these as though they were saturated fatty acids. Look for products that are labelled high in unsaturates.

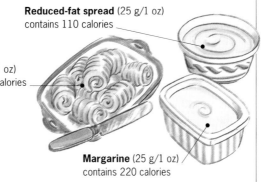

Reduced-fat spread (25 g/1 oz) contains 110 calories

Butter (25 g/1 oz) contains 220 calories

SPREADING FAT
Butter and margarine are both 81 per cent fat. Low-fat spreads, however, may contain as little as five per cent fat. The low percentage of fat is usually achieved by adding water to the spread.

Margarine (25 g/1 oz) contains 220 calories

Fat molecules
The majority of the body's fatty acids are large compounds called triglycerides: three fatty acids linked to a molecule of glycerol (an organic compound). The body's tissues assemble and disassemble triglycerides as needed.

Many triglycerides travel in the body and are stored in the fat depots, such as the upper arm and abdomen, until they are used for fuel.

---

fat stored around the body's organs helps to support and to protect them. The fat layer under the skin acts as a kind of thermal blanket that helps to keep the body warm. Furthermore, fats are an excellent source of energy, storable for future use.

The body can manufacture most types of fatty acids from excess calories eaten in the form of carbohydrates and proteins, but it cannot manufacture them all. Two substances that scientists call essential fatty acids must come from the foods you eat. These two – linoleic acid and linolenic acid –occur naturally in vegetable oils, seeds, nuts, and oily fish. They make up the membranes of each of the trillions of cells in the body and are essential for the synthesis of hormone-like substances called prostaglandins.

If you are to keep healthy, you need to understand more about how fatty foods work in the body, what are the different types of fats found in foods and which foods contain which fats. Then you will be able to choose the kinds of foods that will benefit your body and avoid those that could cause you problems.

THE DIFFERENT FATS
All fats contain fatty acids, which may be saturated or unsaturated. The difference lies in the types of molecules that make them up and the way that these molecules are arranged (see diagram, opposite). The molecules of a saturated fatty acid all contain a full complement of hydrogen atoms. This is what makes them 'saturated'. In contrast, the molecules of unsaturated fatty acids have fewer hydrogen atoms. A high intake of saturated fats can lead to heart disease, but unsaturated fats have a protective effect.

It is possible to distinguish between saturated and unsaturated fats if you bear in mind that saturated fats, including saturated oils, are solid at room temperature, while unsaturated fats are liquid. Saturated fats are found mainly in animal products, such as meat and dairy foods, but also in tropical oils, for example, palm oil, coconut oil and cocoa butter.

Unsaturated fats occur in two forms, polyunsaturated and monounsaturated, and are found in vegetable oils. Olive, peanut, sesame and rapeseed oils contain mostly monounsaturated fats; soya bean, corn, cottonseed, safflower and sunflower oils are mainly made up of polyunsaturated fats. Polyunsaturated fats contain linoleic and linolenic acids, the essential fatty acids that cannot be made by the body.

HOW MUCH FAT DO YOU NEED?
To maintain optimum health, a mature adult requires a minimum quantity of fat – 30 grams per day – 4 grams of which should contain the essential fatty acids that are found in polyunsaturated fats and oils. Thirty grams of fat per day may sound like a large amount but, in fact, it is far less than the average daily intake of most people in Britain. Since every gram of fat provides

Invisible fats
Unfortunately, much of the fat you eat is not visible. Foods like biscuits and pastries are loaded with 'invisible' fats. To avoid these hidden fats, read the label on the packets before buying them. The fat content and the percentage of saturated fat should be clearly marked.

APPEALING LOOK
Manufacturers add fats to biscuits and pastries to make them taste and look better. Coconut oil sprayed on water biscuits, for example, gives them a crisp outer coating and a glossy appearance.

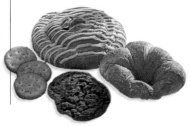

Garlic bread

To accompany a meal, forget butter-soaked garlic bread. Prepare this Mediterranean food the way the Italians do – with olive oil. Then add extra flavour with fresh herbs.

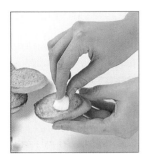

1 *Slice and lightly toast crusty French or Italian bread and rub the rough surfaces of the toast with a cut garlic clove.*

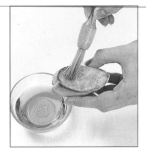

2 *Brush the bread, on one side only, with a little extra-virgin olive oil.*

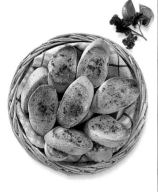

3 *Sprinkle chopped fresh herbs, such as parsley, over the bread and serve at once.*

COMPARISON OF DIETARY FATS

The chart below shows the proportions of saturated, monounsaturated and polyunsaturated fatty acids in various cooking fats. Also shown are the levels of linoleic and linolenic essential fatty acids, which are found in polyunsaturated fat.

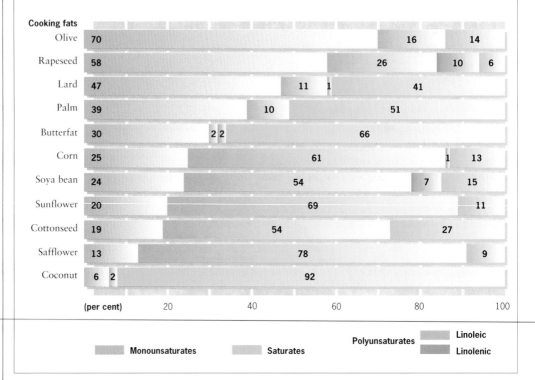

Cooking fats	Monounsaturates	Linoleic	Linolenic	Saturates
Olive	70	16		14
Rapeseed	58	26	10	6
Lard	47	11	1	41
Palm	39	10		51
Butterfat	30	2	2	66
Corn	25	61	1	13
Soya bean	24	54	7	15
Sunflower	20	69		11
Cottonseed	19	54		27
Safflower	13	78		9
Coconut	6	2		92

(per cent) 20 40 60 80 100

Monounsaturates   Saturates   Polyunsaturates — Linoleic / Linolenic

nine calories, 30 grams of fat amount to 270 calories, between 13 and 14 per cent of the daily calorie intake for an adult (about 2000 calories). However, the average adult in Britain gets about 42 per cent of the calories in his or her diet from fat – about 840 calories a day. Most people, therefore, are eating almost three times as much fat as they need. Health authorities in Great Britain now recommend that the intake of fat be reduced to no more than 30 per cent of calories, or about 600 calories a day.

HOW CAN YOU CUT DOWN ON FATS?

Four easy, immediate steps that will reduce your fat intake are trimming all visible fat from meat, switching to low-fat dairy products, spreading butter or margarine more thinly and using low-fat cooking methods, such as steaming or stir-frying, instead of roasting or frying. Next, you should limit your fat intake by eating less butter, eggs, cheese and other dairy products, as well as red meat and even chicken. These foods are high in saturated fats, the culprits of heart disease. If you cannot face the complete exclusion of meats from your life, use cooking techniques that promote the removal of the fat. A meat-based sauce, soup or stew, for instance, can be cooked a day ahead and stored overnight in the refrigerator, to allow the fat to rise to the top of the dish and solidify for easy removal.

Vegetarians, in general, eat a diet that is likely to be lower in fat than a standard diet, since vegetables and grains are virtually free of cholesterol (see p. 56) and are low in fat. But even a meatless diet may include undesirable elements, for example, full-fat dairy products. A dish of macaroni cheese made with a sauce based on butter, full-fat milk and Cheddar cheese can create as much havoc in fat count as a breakfast of bacon and eggs.

Consuming low-fat dairy products such as skimmed milk allows you to reduce the amount of fat in your diet without losing the protein that is in milk products. Snack foods and desserts are often high in fat, but you do not need to give up either completely to lower your fat intake. Instead, change the types of foods you eat. Cut out biscuits, cakes and crisps as much as possible. These 'treats' are especially unhealthy since they contain tropical oils and a great deal of hydrogenated fat (see box on page 51), both of which are highly saturated. Fruit and fruit-based desserts are low-fat, healthier dessert choices, as are sandwiches or popcorn for snacks.

EATING THE 'GOOD' FATS

Another way to reduce your intake of saturated fats is to substitute monounsaturated olive oil or polyunsaturated oil such as sunflower oil for butter and tropical oils in cooking. Although these oils have as many calories, gram for gram, as saturated oils they have a different effect on cholesterol metabolism – a major factor in coronary artery disease (see p. 110).

DID YOU KNOW?

Pork and beef both have a reputation as fatty meats. But while some pork products such as chopped ham are indeed high in fat, lean ham, at five per cent fat, contains less fat than lean beef. Rump steak, for example, is seven per cent fat.

Certain fish oils are particularly beneficial. They contain a class of essential fatty acids known as omega-3 fatty acids, which are polyunsaturates that have been shown to lower cholesterol and reduce the blood's ability to clot and clog up the arteries. Cold water ocean fish, such as mackerel, herring, tuna, sardines and salmon are all rich in this type of oil. Experts recommend that you eat these fish twice a week.

Can you eat too little fat?

Although most people believe that they are eating too much fat, some people are actually not eating enough. People on strict weight-loss diets can be at risk of eating too little fat, as can people who eat a highly fat-restricted diet based heavily on complex carbohydrates. Everyone needs some fat to survive (about 30 grams per day). Some experts believe that anorexia and bulimia sufferers may become infertile because they do not eat the fats necessary for normal hormone production.

Most of the dietary recommendations for middle-aged people should not be applied to young children, who have high energy requirements and need fat to meet their needs. A change to low-fat products, such as skimmed milk, can mean that a child's hunger is satisfied before energy needs have been met. Children should, therefore, drink whole milk until they are two years old.

REDUCED-FAT EATING

HIGH FAT	HEALTHIER FAT
POTATOES	
Deep-fat frying	Cook 'oven' chips in unsaturated oil. Blot chips on kitchen paper.
POULTRY	
Skin on	Remove skin before cooking.
Butter baste	Baste with stock.
MEAT	
Heavily marbled cuts	Choose lean cuts; trim fat off meat.
Pan gravy	Skim fat off gravy.
PASTA	
Served with meaty sauces or creamy sauces	Make vegetable-based sauces. Toss pasta in a little olive oil and herbs.
FISH	
Fried	Poach, bake in foil or paper, steam or microwave.
STEWS	
Meat-based	Trim fat off meat, skim fat off stew, use more vegetables and pulses. Use minimum fat to fry meat or vegetables or use olive oil for frying.
CHEESE TOPPINGS	
Full-fat cheese	Use low-fat cheese or breadcrumb toppings flavoured with herbs and garlic.
GARLIC BREAD	
Butter	Use olive oil; spread with pastry brush.

The Naturopath

Naturopathy is a system of health care that uses natural measures, particularly diet, to restore and promote your body's self-healing processes. Taking a holistic approach, a naturopath is able to identify and treat the causes of illness.

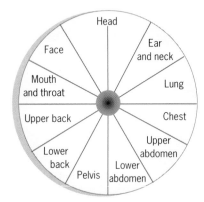

IRIS DIAGNOSIS
Some naturopaths use careful inspection of the eye as a diagnostic aid. The iris (the coloured part of the eye) is believed to have reflex connections with other organs and tissues in the body. Changes in the texture of these zones may reveal information about the health of the related organs.

Naturopaths may advise or apply treatments that differ from those of conventional medicine, but are, nevertheless, complementary to the services available from your doctor.

What sort of treatment does a naturopath give?

Instead of relying on drugs, naturopaths use various therapies to capitalise on the body's natural healing ability. Dietary therapy, fasting, hydrotherapy, massage and osteopathy – one or several of these therapies may be used to treat an individual's ailment.

What sort of illnesses can a naturopath cure or alleviate?

Naturopaths treat a wide range of illnesses, both acute and chronic, as well as infections. For acute illnesses, such as colds, coughs and gastroenteritis, the naturopath will suggest safe and effective ways of relieving the symptoms without the need to resort to antibiotics or other suppressive drugs. The naturopath will apply similar treatments to alleviate chronic illnesses, such as rheumatism, arthritis and asthma.

Why would I consult a naturopath?

If you want to take more personal responsibility for your health and prefer to use natural treatments whenever possible, you might decide to seek the advice of a naturopath.

The naturopath tailors his or her advice to your individual needs and will usually suggest modifications to your diet for a few days, in conjunction with other treatments such as herbal remedies.

How does a naturopath decide which treatment to give?

At your first visit, the naturopath will ask you about any health problems, your diet, work, exercise, lifestyle and personal history. All these elements will be taken into consideration when establishing your health programme.

The naturopath is trained in basic medical sciences, such as anatomy, physiology and diagnosis. This training enables him or her to carry out a full medical examination and

Origins

Although the term *naturopathy* was not adopted until the end of the 19th century, this system of medicine dates back to Hippocrates, whose recommendations more than 2000 years ago included the maxim 'Let food be your medicine and let your medicine be your food'.

In the 19th and early 20th century, pioneers such as Stanley Lief in England, Max Bircher-Benner in Switzerland and Henry Lindlahr in the United States, all ran residential clinics at which patients were able to fast and undergo physical therapy and water treatments to tackle a wide variety of ailments. These forerunners of modern scientific naturopathy were determined advocates of diets low in

fats, salt and refined foods – diets that are now widely endorsed by health experts around the world.

FATHER OF WESTERN MEDICINE
The Greek physician, Hippocrates (c.460–c.370 BC), maintained that the body could heal itself with the aid of natural cures, such as a good diet.

to use information gained from the initial consultation not only for normal diagnostic purposes but also to assess your vitality and potential for better health. Many naturopaths also use other investigations, such as blood, sweat and hair analysis, to check your levels of the minerals and trace elements that are essential for a healthy body. Some naturopaths may also use iris diagnosis (see opposite).

How does naturopathy help infectious diseases?

Naturopaths regard many acute illnesses, especially those that are accompanied by a fever, as a sign of the self-healing mechanisms at work. As your immune system starts to overcome the infection, your body temperature rises, either locally with inflammation, or more generally with a fever. Naturopaths believe that this must be allowed to take its course without suppressing the symptoms. In this situation, they recommend fasting or, in cases where this may not be appropriate,

a restricted diet, such as fresh fruit only for two or three days. This allows your body to rid itself of the toxic compounds associated with the infection. You may also be shown how to use cold compresses to assist detoxification, regulate temperature and increase your immune response.

How does naturopathy help chronic diseases?

When chronic degenerative diseases, such as arthritis, have taken their toll, the body's self-healing capacity may be limited, but naturopathic treatment can still help to keep the patient more comfortable and reduce dependence on pain-relieving drugs. Diet control is often a major part of this management.

For patients with heart and circulatory problems, the naturopath is able to give guidance on how to substitute unsaturated fats in the diet for those that are not easily digested. Advice on exercise and relaxation is also important for dealing with these disorders.

CHECKING YOUR HEALTH
The naturopath will usually carry out a full medical examination, including taking your blood pressure.

How can I find a naturopath?

You may consult a naturopath without referral from a medical practitioner, although it is preferable that your doctor should know that you are seeking such advice.

Most naturopaths are in private practice and may be seen by appointment. Some practitioners work in residential clinics where a range of treatments, such as spa baths, are available to patients.

In the United Kingdom, naturopaths who are registered with the General Council and Register of Naturopaths (GCRN) have undergone a four year full-time training. The GCRN publishes a directory of qualified practitioners and is based at Frazer House, 6 Netherhall Gardens, London NW3 5RR.

WHAT YOU CAN DO AT HOME

Nearly everyone experiences an attack of vomiting and diarrhoea at some time. This may be caused by tainted food or gastric 'flu'. In either case, the following diet may help (seek the advice of your general practitioner before undertaking this diet if you have any medical disorder, such as diabetes or epilepsy).

TIME	DIET
First 24 hours	Drink one tumbler of unsweetened apple juice or mineral water every two or three hours. This allows the stomach and intestines to clear fermented matter and irritants.
Second day	Breakfast – a little low-fat yoghurt. Lunch – a dish of finely grated or puréed apple. Evening meal – if you feel better, have a bowl of vegetable soup.
Third day	Have fruit and yoghurt for breakfast; soup or steamed vegetables with a savoury dish of brown rice for lunch and dinner.

THE DANGERS OF A HIGH-FAT DIET

Many international studies have indicated a link between high-fat diets and increased death rates from hypertension, heart disease, stroke and cancer.

Foods that raise cholesterol

Despite all the attention that cholesterol has received, many people still do not know which foods contain the fats that produce it.

Cholesterol-raising saturated fats are found mainly in foods derived from animals – meat, poultry, shellfish and dairy products. Coconut and palm oils, although derived from plants, are also high in saturated fats. Only ten per cent of your fat calories should come from saturated fats.

HIGH-FAT FOODS
A high intake of full-fat dairy products and fatty meats will raise your level of 'bad' cholesterol – LDLs – and increase your risk of heart disease. But a fatty food like avocado provides unsaturated fat, which does not harm the arteries.

The connection between a high-fat diet and life-threatening diseases such as hypertension, heart disease, stroke and cancer centres on a waxy substance known as cholesterol. Although naturally occurring cholesterol is found in some foods, particularly offal and egg yolks, most of the cholesterol in the body is manufactured in the liver and other tissues from ingested saturated fats.

There are three types of lipoprotein (protein-covered fat particles) in the bloodstream that transport cholesterol throughout the body. Two of these lipoproteins are harmful if excessive, while the third seems to have a beneficial effect on your arteries.

Low-density lipoprotein (LDL) and very-low-density lipoprotein (VLDL) tend to stick to the lining of the arteries and appear to increase in relation to the amount of saturated fat a person eats. However, high-density lipoprotein (HDL) has the capacity to dissolve existing cholesterol residue in the arteries and scrub it from the blood vessel walls as it passes. Levels of protective HDL cholesterol are increased by a low-fat diet that contains a good supply of fruit and vegetables. Other factors that increase this 'good' cholesterol are exercising regularly, drinking small quantities of alcohol, particularly red wine, and eating fish such as tuna, mackerel, salmon or herring, which are rich in omega-3 fatty acids.

CHOLESTEROL AND DISEASE

When people eat more saturated fats than they need, cholesterol production within the body increases, and excess cholesterol ends up in the bloodstream where it accumulates on the walls of the arteries.

Over the years, the arterial walls can become lined with these fatty deposits, or plaques. The condition – a thickening and stiffening of the walls of the arteries – is known as atherosclerosis. The thicker walls means that the passageway for blood is narrower – which increases blood pressure.

High blood pressure, or hypertension, is a major health risk. When arteries are narrowed, blood must be pushed more forcefully through them, placing the walls under additional strain. They can begin to weaken and form bulges, known as aneurisms. If these bulges rupture, they may cause a

HIGH FAT AND CANCER

Cancer is a very complex disease with many causes, but certain types have been associated with diet. Bile acids in the colon that can turn cells cancerous are stimulated by fat. Fat is also known to act as a fuel promoting tumour growth. Recent research indicates that eating too much fat can depress the immune system's tumour surveillance mechanism.

Despite these findings, the evidence remains controversial and the link between diet and cancer is yet to be completely proven. Some scientists now believe that oxidised fat and cholesterol may be the culprits and that high levels of antioxidants (see p. 94), which come from fruits, vegetables and vegetable oils, may play a protective role.

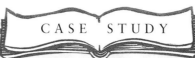

High Blood Cholesterol

Cholesterol is a normal component of blood, but when blood cholesterol levels are permanently raised, the individual becomes susceptible to a number of diseases. A high cholesterol level may be caused by various factors, among them poor diet, alcohol abuse and genetic disease. Sufferers may need to make several modifications to their diet to control this condition.

At the age of 40, Barbara Becker spends most of her time caring for her husband and two teenage sons. Recently a friend pointed out that Barbara had white rings in her eyes, around the edges of her irises. These, and some little lumps she has noticed on the back of her right hand, prompted her to go to see her doctor. She was shocked to learn that these rings and lumps are indications of dangerously high blood cholesterol levels. Barbara's doctor explained that permanently high levels of blood cholesterol contribute to heart attack, high blood pressure, stroke, and sudden death, but that through proper medication, a low-fat diet and giving up cigarettes, her medical problems can be controlled. He also suggested that her form of high cholesterol was probably inherited.

WHAT SHOULD BARBARA DO?

Barbara must take the medication prescribed by her doctor to control her blood cholesterol levels, and she should have regular check-ups. She should also take the precaution of ensuring that her sons have their blood cholesterol levels checked, not just once, but every five years.

Barbara and her doctor should agree on a diet that will help her to reduce her intake of saturated fats and cholesterol and increase her intake of soluble fibre (see p. 46). She not only needs to educate herself about low-fat cooking, but she must also alert those around her to the dangers in their eating habits not only at home but also outside it.

Barbara needs to find behaviour modification techniques that will help her to give up smoking. Her local hospital will provide advice.

HEALTH
A diet high in saturated fats and an addiction to cigarettes have added to the risks already existing with an inherited tendency towards high cholesterol levels.

FAMILY
A genetic disposition to high levels of cholesterol may have been inherited by a sufferer's children as well as herself.

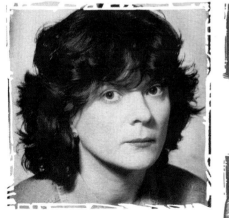

Action Plan

HEALTH
Seek advice on a changed dietary pattern. Go for more regular check-ups. Stop smoking now.

FAMILY
Make sure the boys' cholesterol levels are tested. Also try to get the whole family more involved in their health and teach them about eating more sensibly.

HOW THINGS TURNED OUT FOR BARBARA

Barbara's doctor referred her to a dietitian, who assessed her current eating pattern and lifestyle. She recommended a balanced, reduced-fat diet with several servings of fruit and vegetables every day to help Barbara eat more healthily. Barbara's improved diet gave her more energy, but she has gone back to preparing and eating more of the quick foods and frozen pies her family enjoys. She finds this worrying, since the boys' cholesterol levels did turn out to be higher than normal. Another trip to the dietitian has been planned, this time with the boys, to get more ideas about changing their diet. Smoking is still a problem, but she is now down to three cigarettes a day.

LOWERING CHOLESTEROL LEVELS

Changing the types of foods you eat can help you to keep your overall cholesterol levels low or reduce them if they have become too high and can raise the levels of 'good' cholesterol – HDLs.

▶ *Increase the amount of fruits and vegetables in your diet, whether fresh, frozen or canned.*

▶ *Eat more foods containing water soluble fibre, such as pulses and oat bran (see p. 46).*

BENEFICIAL FOODS
Salmon, pulses, fruits, vegetables and red wine actually lower 'bad' cholesterol and reduce the blood's ability to clot and clog up the arteries.

stroke or cardiac arrest. Strokes occur when arteries in the brain rupture, leaking blood into the surrounding tissue, while the heart may stop if its blood supply is interfered with. Even if such severe consequences do not occur, high blood pressure can cause damage to the kidneys or the retina.

Large-scale international studies connecting eating habits with patterns of illness have tended to confirm the link between a diet high in saturated fat and heart disease. In Japan and the Mediterranean countries people eat a diet low in saturated fat and they are consequently less likely to develop heart disease than citizens of northern European countries or the United States, who eat higher amounts of saturated fat. They also eat more fish, which are low in saturated fat, and less meat. In Mediterranean countries people eat a high amount of fat, but it is mainly olive oil, not butter.

The health and eating habits of the Inuits of Greenland confirms the importance of the type of fat eaten. Although the Inuits eat a very high-fat diet, heart disease and stroke are virtually unknown. The reason for this anomaly is that the fats they eat come from fatty fish and seal blubber and are mostly unsaturated. These foods also contain large amounts of omega-3 fatty acids, which lower levels of 'bad' cholesterol (LDLs), dilate the blood vessels (which helps to relieve pressure), and counteract the formation of blood clots.

International studies have also shown a high correlation between the incidence of breast cancer and the level of dietary fat. In Europe

LOW-FAT OR LOW-CALORIE?

Reports concerning the links between dietary fat and major illnesses have stimulated considerable public demand for foods containing little or no fat, particularly among dieters. But fat-free products do not guarantee weight loss, and if they form too large a part of your diet, they may even be harmful.

Fat-free products can only help you to lose weight if you are eating fewer calories than you burn up. Being fat-free is not the same as being calorie-free. Carbohydrates and proteins in food contain calories, and eating excessive amounts of fat-free foods in the mistaken belief that they will not make you fat will certainly not help to make you slim.

Even if you are dieting, you should be sure to eat some fats or oils every day. Dressing salads with a little olive oil, adding seeds and soya bean products to your meals and eating oily fish two or three times a week may cost you some calories, but they are a good investment for long-term health.

and the United States, where the percentage of fat in the diet is high, the rate of breast cancer is also high; in Japan and other countries where less fat is eaten, the rates for this cancer are lower.

Colo-rectal cancer is also most prevalent in economically developed countries, where individuals eat a diet that is high in fat and low in fibre.

LOWER FAT SUBSTITUTES

SUBSTITUTE	INSTEAD OF	SAVE
2 egg whites	1 whole egg	5 g fat
25 g (1 oz) low-fat mozzarella	25 g (1 oz) Cheddar cheese	4 g fat
25 g (1 oz) cottage cheese	25 g (1 oz) cream cheese	9 g fat
2 slices bread with low-fat spread	2 slices bread with butter	11 g fat
25 g (1oz) extra-lean roast ham	25 g (1oz) hard salami	12 g fat
1 pork chop, lean only, grilled	1 pork chop, lean and fat, grilled	19 g fat
115 g (4 oz) tuna in brine	115 g (4 oz) tuna in oil	7 g fat
1 x 115 g (4 oz) baked potato	1 x 100 g (3½ oz) portion chips	14 g fat
1 banana	1 iced doughnut	13 g fat
55 g (2 oz) sorbet	55 g (2 oz) ice cream	10 g fat

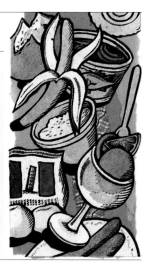

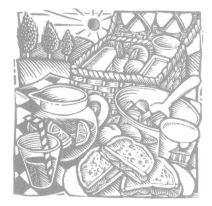

VITAMINS AND MINERALS

*Although needed by the body in only tiny
amounts, vitamins and minerals are essential
for good health. A balanced diet can provide
ample amounts of these nutrients, but poor eating
habits can deprive you of the vitamins and minerals
you need. While supplements can give you the
nutrients you should have, in the long run it is
much better to eat sensibly, choose foods wisely
and prepare, cook and store them properly.*

MICRONUTRIENTS

Peanuts – 42 g (1½ oz) contain 6 mg of niacin

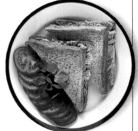

A tuna sandwich contains 6 mg of niacin

SOURCES OF NIACIN (VITAMIN B₃)
A sandwich containing 25 g (1 oz) tuna provides as much of the B vitamin niacin as 42 g (1½ oz) of peanuts.

Vitamins are life-sustaining substances that humans need to keep their bodies working efficiently. Minerals have an equally vital role in developing and maintaining the body's functions.

Unlike the macronutrients – proteins, carbohydrates and fats – vitamins do not provide energy or serve as building materials. Instead, they enable the body to function efficiently by regulating biochemical processes such as growth metabolism, cellular reproduction, digestion and the oxidation of blood.

There are 13 recognised vitamins, and these are classified into two groups, water-soluble and fat-soluble. Water-soluble vitamins, which include the B complex group and C, remain for no more than three days in various body tissues; therefore they need to be replenished daily. They are absorbed through the intestine into the bloodstream and any excess that the body does not need passes out in urine. If your diet is severely lacking in these vitamins, deficiency symptoms can occur within weeks.

Four fat-soluble vitamins – A, D, E and K – are absorbed through the intestine with dietary fats and (except vitamin K) are stored in the liver and fatty tissue. They can be stockpiled for periods that, depending on quantity, can be as long as a year (or more in the case of vitamin A), so you do not need to consume large quantities of them every day. In fact, excessive amounts of fat-soluble vitamins in the diet can be harmful.

WATER-SOLUBLE VITAMINS

There are eight members of the B-complex group. Each has separate functions, but they all are essential for efficient metabolism – the process by which the body converts food into tissue or uses it to produce energy. B vitamins play a major role in the body's production of energy, working with enzymes – body substances that break down foods – to convert carbohydrates and fats into fuel for the body. They are also necessary for the functioning of the nervous and immune systems.

Thiamin (B₁) aids the release of energy from food, and from all body cells including the brain and nerve cells and the muscles. Riboflavin (B₂) helps to liberate energy from carbohydrates and fats.

Niacin (B₃) is also crucial for energy release and protein metabolism – conversion of protein to substances of use to the body – and the production of certain hormones. Unlike thiamin and riboflavin, which can be obtained only from food, niacin can be partially synthesised within the body from the amino acid tryptophan. Since not enough can be made, however, dietary sources are also needed.

THE ROLE OF THE LIVER

The liver, which produces bile, a digestive juice, plays an active role in breaking down fats in foods. This allows fat-soluble vitamins and other nutrients to be absorbed through the small intestine, converting them for use in the body.

The liver is also a storehouse for nutrients, such as minerals and three of the fat-soluble vitamins – A, D and E.

Gall bladder stores bile secreted by the liver. It releases bile when needed

Bile duct drains bile into the intestine

Oesophagus

Stomach

Duodenum

Small intestine

Liver

Colon

ABSORBING FAT-SOLUBLE VITAMINS
The intestine is lined with layers of cells (villi) through which fat-soluble vitamins pass into the bloodstream. Excess vitamins are carried to the liver for storage.

B₁₂ AND THE INTRINSIC FACTOR

Cells in the stomach lining secrete an enzyme called the intrinsic factor. This binds with vitamin B_{12}, allowing it to be absorbed into the bloodstream from the intestinal tract.

People who lack this enzyme must have vitamin B_{12} injected into the bloodstream under the supervision of a doctor or clinical nutritionist.

THE STOMACH
The wall of the stomach consists of three layers of smooth muscle. Its inner lining is made up of cells that secrete gastric juice, which contains the intrinsic factor.

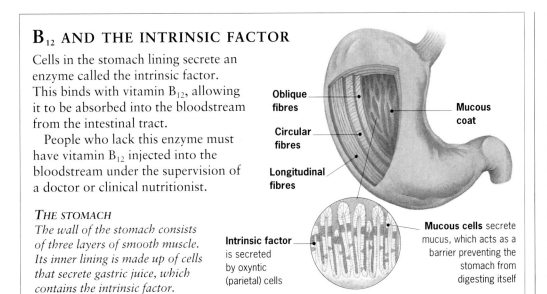

Oblique fibres

Circular fibres

Longitudinal fibres

Mucous coat

Mucous cells secrete mucus, which acts as a barrier preventing the stomach from digesting itself

Intrinsic factor is secreted by oxyntic (parietal) cells

(see p. 51)

Pantothenic acid, another member of the B group, also enables the body to obtain energy from foods and helps the body to manufacture some important hormones.

Vitamin B_6 helps the body to absorb and use proteins. The more high-protein foods you eat, such as meat, the more foods containing vitamin B_6 you will need. Vitamin B_6 also helps to maintain the central nervous system and, along with folic acid and B_{12}, helps to form haemoglobin, the oxygen-carrying pigment in red blood cells. Vitamin B_6 plays a role in the metabolism of essential fatty acids (see p. 51), and is involved in more than 80 biochemical reactions.

Vitamin B_{12} is essential for the production of healthy red blood cells and for preventing anaemia. In the manufacture of red blood cells, vitamin B_{12} acts in conjunction with folic acid, both of which play a vital part in the synthesis of genetic material. It also helps the nervous system to function smoothly and assists in the metabolism of amino acids. Unlike other B vitamins, the only natural sources of B_{12} are animal products and some fermented foods.

Biotin, another water-soluble vitamin, helps the body to utilise essential fatty acids and is necessary for releasing energy from carbohydrates and proteins as well as fat.

Vitamin C
A major role in healing wounds and burns is played by vitamin C, which also aids the absorption of iron from grains and leafy vegetables. Vitamin C helps to produce collagen, the basis of connective tissue, which holds together the various structures of the body. Contrary to popular belief, studies have not yet supported the claim that large doses of vitamin C can ward off completely or cure the common cold. Research suggests, however, that it does help to reduce the cold's duration. Vitamin C is also a potent antioxidant, neutralising free radicals. These are unstable molecules, that if

PRESERVING VITAMINS

Vitamins are very fragile nutrients that are easily destroyed during storage and cooking. Here are a few tips to help you to get the most from food.

▶ *Store foods in a cool, dark area because light accelerates vitamin loss, particularly of vitamins A, D and B_2.*

▶ *Rinse fruit and vegetables under cold, running water. Do not soak them because the vitamins will leach into the water.*

▶ *Microwave, pressure cook or steam vegetables in a small amount of water. Otherwise the vitamins will pass into the cooking water.*

NUTRIENT COMBINATIONS

Particular vitamins and minerals, eaten in tandem, will work more effectively in the body. Some are found in one food alone, others in combinations of foods.

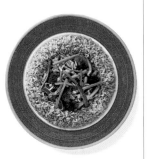

Vitamin D and calcium – the flesh of sardines contains vitamin D, and their bones calcium. A good level of vitamin D aids the body to use calcium more effectively

Vitamin E and essential fatty acids – sunflower seeds add vitamin E, which protects against oxidation of essential fatty acids provided by olive oil in a stir-fry

Vitamin B_{12} and folic acid – a good source of vitamin B_{12}, eggs can be combined with the folic acid in spinach to form new cells in the body

Vitamin C and iron – tomato sauce provides vitamin C, which helps the absorption of iron from rice and vegetables

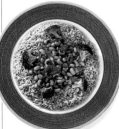

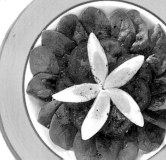

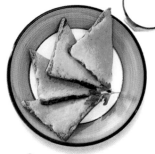

An orange
contains 54 mg
of calcium

Milk – 225 ml (8 fl oz)
contain 297 mg
of calcium

SOURCES OF CALCIUM
You can meet three-quarters of your daily calcium needs simply by eating two slices of wholemeal toast, 55 g (2 oz) of cheese, a glass of milk and an orange.

unchecked contribute to heart disease and cancers and are associated with the ageing process (see p. 94). It has also been demonstrated that vitamin C helps to block the formation of cancer-causing substances called nitrosamines, which are formed in the stomach from nitrites in foods.

FAT-SOLUBLE VITAMINS
Vitamin A (retinol), is essential both for good vision and for the manufacture of rhodopsin, or visual purple. This is a light-sensitive pigment in the retina – the part of the eye that reacts to light. Vitamin A also helps to form healthy skin and mucous membranes, such as the linings of the nose and digestive system, and is essential for the proper functioning of the liver. Growth and development also rely on an adequate intake of vitamin A. Beta carotene, which is converted into vitamin A in the body, is a powerful antioxidant, mopping up free radicals before damage can occur. Carotenes are so called because they were first isolated

from carrots. About 35 of more than 6000 carotenes in nature can be partially converted by the body in the intestinal wall to vitamin A. The remainder of the carotenes are absorbed directly into the body.

Vitamin D (cholecalciferol) is vital for the development and maintenance of bones and teeth, and aids in the absorption and metabolism of calcium and phosphorus. Nicknamed the 'sunshine vitamin', it is made by the skin when the skin is exposed to the ultraviolet light in sunshine. It is also found in a number of foods, particularly fortified milk.

Vitamin E (tocopherol) is a potent antioxidant. Along with vitamin C and the carotenes, it is important for dissipating free radicals (see p. 94) and protecting essential fatty acids from oxidation. Recent research suggests that vitamin E helps to protect against cancer and heart disease by limiting the production of free radicals.

Vitamin K is essential for producing the substances in the liver that promote blood clotting. It is found in a wide range of foods

RECOMMENDED DAILY ALLOWANCE OF VITAMINS

AGES	A μg	D μg	C mg	B_1 mg	B_2 mg	B_3 mg	B_6 mg	FOLIC ACID μg	B_{12} μg
INFANTS									
To 6 mths	350	8.5	25	0.2	0.4	3	0.2	50	0.3
6 mths–1 yr	350	7	25	0.3	0.4	5	0.4	50	0.4
CHILDREN									
1–3 yrs	400	7	30	0.5	0.6	8	0.7	70	0.5
4–6	500	–	30	0.7	0.8	11	0.9	100	0.8
7–10	500	–	30	0.7	1	12	1	150	1
MALES									
11–14	600	–	35	0.9	1.2	15	1.2	200	1.2
15–18	700	–	40	1.1	1.3	18	1.5	200	1.5
19–22	700	–	40	1	1.3	17	1.4	200	1.5
23–50	700	–	40	1	1.3	17	1.4	200	1.5
51 & over	700	–	40	0.9	1.3	16	1.4	200	1.5
FEMALES									
11–14	600	–	35	0.7	1.1	12	1	200	1.2
15–18	600	–	40	0.8	1.1	14	1.2	200	1.5
19–22	600	–	40	0.8	1.1	13	1.2	200	1.5
23–50	600	–	40	0.8	1.1	13	1.2	200	1.5
51 & over	600	–	40	0.8	1.1	12	1.2	200	1.5
Pregnant	+100	10	+10	+0.1	+0.3	no extra	no extra	+100	no extra
Nursing	+350	10	+30	+0.2	+0.5	+2	no extra	+60	+0.5

mg= milligrams   µg= micrograms

Source: Dietary Reference Values for Food Energy and Nutrients for the United Kingdom © Crown copyright 1991

and, because it is also made by intestinal bacteria, most people have some supply. Newborn babies, however, are born with low stores of the vitamin and are at risk of haemorrhaging. Vitamin K is now routinely administered to all babies.

THE MINERALS

Like vitamins, minerals are vital for the body's well-being – they are essential components of critical enzymes that help the body to break down food.

Calcium, phosphorus, magnesium, potassium, sodium and chloride are known as macrominerals: they are needed in fairly large quantities by the body.

Calcium is indispensable for building and maintaining strong bones and teeth. About 99 per cent of the body's calcium is found in the bones and teeth, with the remaining 1 per cent being distributed in the cells, blood and bodily fluids. Everybody needs a good supply of calcium throughout life to sustain bone density and strength, but the greater the bone density early in life, the less the risk of bones becoming porous in old age (see p. 69).

The calcium in cells performs a variety of functions, including ensuring the proper functioning of the nerves and muscles and normal clotting of the blood. Vitamin D is required for calcium absorption, but studies have shown that exercising will also speed up this process.

Magnesium is essential for the proper functioning of nerves and muscles and for maintaining bone structure. It also aids fat metabolism, regulation of body temperature and protein synthesis.

Phosphorus works closely with calcium and magnesium to build and maintain bones and teeth. It also plays a role in releasing energy from carbohydrates and transporting fats around the body.

Potassium, one of the body's most abundant minerals, is crucial for controlling water balance in the body's tissues and cells. It also helps to regulate blood pressure.

Strawberries – provide 0.6 mg of iron

Spinach – provides 2 mg of iron

Cranberry juice – 225 ml (8 fl oz) supplies 0.8 mg of iron

SOURCES OF IRON
A meal consisting of a 115 g (4 oz) steak, 100 g (3½ oz) red kidney beans and the same amount of spinach, 85 g (3 oz) bulghur wheat, 140 g (5 oz) strawberries and a glass of cranberry juice supplies 13.6 mg of iron.

RECOMMENDED DAILY ALLOWANCE OF MINERALS

AGES	CALCIUM mg	PHOSPHORUS mg	MAGNESIUM mg	IRON mg	ZINC mg	IODINE µg
INFANTS						
To 6 mths	525	400	60	4.3	4	60
6 mths–1 yr	525	400	80	7.8	5	60
CHILDREN						
1–3 yrs	350	270	85	6.9	5	70
4–6	450	350	120	6.1	6.5	100
7–10	550	450	200	8.7	7	110
MALES						
11–14	1000	775	280	11.3	9	130
15–18	1000	775	300	11.3	9.5	140
19–22	700	550	300	8.7	9.5	140
23–50	700	550	300	8.7	9.5	140
51 & over	700	550	300	8.7	9.5	140
FEMALES						
11–14	800	625	280	14.8	9	130
15–18	800	625	300	14.8	7	140
19–22	700	550	270	14.8	7	140
23–50	700	550	270	14.8	7	140
51 & over	700	550	270	8.7	7	140
Pregnant	no extra	no extra	no extra	no extra	no extra	no extra
Nursing	+550	+440	+50	no extra	+2.5	no extra

mg= milligrams   µg= micrograms

Source: Dietary Reference Values for Food Energy and Nutrients for the United Kingdom © Crown copyright 1991

Sodium and chloride work as partners with potassium to balance the body's fluids. Sodium is also essential for nerve activity.

Iron, zinc, iodine, manganese, selenium, chromium, copper and fluoride are all trace elements. Although the body needs smaller amounts of these minerals than of the so-called macrominerals, they have an equally vital role in the functioning of the body.

Iron is essential for the formation of haemoglobin, the red pigment in the bloodstream that transports oxygen from the lungs to all the cells of the body. It is also an important component of many enzymes.

Zinc is necessary for normal mental, physical and reproductive development, hair and skin growth, wound healing and insulin production.

VITAMINS – SOURCES AND EFFECTS

There are many tales about the wonderful effects that vitamins can have – and some of them are true. Other claims exaggerate and expand upon the properties of vitamins until we no longer know if a carrot will help us to see in the dark or not. Use the table below to help to discern the difference between myth and reality.

VITAMIN	SOURCES	SAID TO	ACTUALLY IS/DOES
A	Liver, fish (cod and halibut), eggs, dairy products, green and orange vegetables.	Give superhuman sight. Cure cancer. Preserve youthful looks.	Vital to good vision. Important for healthy skin and immunity.
B_1	Wheatgerm, pork and other lean meats, milk, eggs, yeast, dried beans.	Prevent fatigue. Cure depression.	Necessary for functioning of brain, nerve cells and heart.
B_2	Milk, dairy products, eggs, meats, leafy green vegetables, nuts, liver.	Improve vision. Cure baldness.	Required to release energy from foods.
B_3	Peanuts, poultry, meats, milk, eggs, whole grains, liver.	Help schizophrenia. Cure depression.	Maintain healthy skin, nerves and digestive system.
PANTO-THENIC ACID	Eggs, dairy products, fish, cereals, pulses, brewer's yeast.	Ease stress. Return grey hair to normal. Ease allergies.	Essential in the synthesis of many body materials.
B_6	Bananas, wholegrain bread, meats, eggs, dried beans, nuts, chicken, fish, liver.	Help arthritis. Relieve nausea. Act as a tranquilliser. Relieve nervous or muscle disorders.	Important in chemical reactions between proteins and amino acids. Aid formation of red blood cells.
B_{12}	Eggs, shellfish, meats, milk, poultry.	Cure nervous disorders.	Develop red blood cells and maintain the nervous system.
BIOTIN	Eggs, dairy products, liver, cereals.	Help muscle pain. Help cure baldness and dermatitis.	Help to metabolise amino acids, carbohydrates and fats.
FOLIC ACID	Leafy green vegetables, pulses, liver, yeast.	Alleviate mental illness. Prevent birth defects. Cure anaemia.	Act with B_{12} to produce haemoglobin. Important in cell multiplication. Prevent spina bifida in newborn babies.
C	Citrus fruits, strawberries, blackcurrants, tomatoes, melons, potatoes, sweet peppers.	Cure allergies. Cure arthritis. Cure and prevent colds. Prevent atherosclerosis. Prevent certain cancers.	Promote healthy gum, teeth and connective tissue. Aid the healing of wounds. Fight free radicals. Strengthen immune system.
D	Cod liver oil, oily fish, egg yolk, fortified milk and margarines.	Cure arthritis.	Promote strong bones and teeth. Prevent rickets and osteomalacia (softening of the bones).
E	Vegetable oils, sunflower seeds, nuts, wheatgerm, leafy green vegetables.	Improve virility and stamina. Heal burns and scars. Prevent ageing.	Protect tissue against oxidative damage.
K	Leafy green vegetables, soya beans, cereals.		Necessary for normal blood clotting.

Iodine is vital for normal functioning of the thyroid gland, which regulates the body's metabolism, the rate at which the body functions. The mineral also helps to maintain healthy skin, hair and nails.

Manganese aids reproduction, cell function and bone growth and development. Selenium is an important antioxidant and functions as such in conjunction with the vitamins A, C and E. Chromium maintains normal blood sugar levels and is essential for insulin to act properly.

Copper is needed in small quantities by the body to develop red blood cells and facilitate bone synthesis.

Fluoride is vital for the formation and strength of bones and teeth, hardening their crystalline deposits.

MINERALS – SOURCES AND EFFECTS

Great stories are also told about the special properties of minerals. Some of these claims probably arose to encourage children to eat their 'greens'; others have their roots in generations of observation and folk wisdom. But, whatever their origins, the table below will help you to unravel the truth.

MINERAL	SOURCES	SAID TO	ACTUALLY IS/DOES
CALCIUM	Dairy products, dried peas, canned sardines and salmon including bones, leafy green vegetables, oranges.	Build bones and teeth.	Build healthy bones and teeth. Regulate blood clotting and prevent muscle spasms.
CHROMIUM	Brewer's yeast, wheatgerm, cheese.	Help hypoglycaemia. Cure diabetes.	Important for glucose metabolism and insulin production, which are necessary for prevention of diabetes and hypoglycaemia.
COPPER	Liver, kidneys, nuts, cocoa.	Cure anaemia.	Necessary for the formation of red blood cells and absorption of iron.
FLUORIDE	Fluoridated water, canned fish (with bones).	Cause cancer.	Contribute to strong bones and teeth.
IODINE	Seafood, eggs, iodised salt.	Cause anaemia.	Keep skin, hair and nails healthy. Maintain normal thyroid function. Prevent goitre.
IRON	Red meat, liver, eggs, dried beans, leafy green vegetables, molasses.	Control alcoholism and menstrual discomfort. Cure anaemia.	Vital for the production of haemoglobin and myoglobin.
MAGNESIUM	Nuts, bananas, apricots, soya beans.	Cure heart disease. Help with alcoholism and prostate problems. Cure kidney stones.	Regulate heart rhythm. Needed for bone growth.
MANGANESE	Leafy green vegetables, tea.	Cure diabetes. Help fatigue and asthma. Cure sterility.	Necessary for normal cell function, bone growth and reproduction.
POTASSIUM	Bananas, meats, potatoes, oranges, dried fruits.	Cure heart disease. Cure acne and arthritis. Alleviate alcoholism. Heal burns.	Regulate muscle contraction and blood pressure. Control water balance in tissues and cells.
PHOSPHORUS	Dairy products, meats, fish, nuts, whole grains, processed foods.	Cure arthritis. Accelerate children's growth. Reduce stress.	Promote strong teeth and bones. Necessary for energy metabolism.
SELENIUM	Seafood, garlic, tomatoes.	Cure cancer and arthritis.	Fight oxidative cell damage in conjunction with vitamin E.
SODIUM	Table salt, processed foods (for example, bacon, smoked fish).	Lower fever. Protect against cramp. Raise blood pressure.	Balance water in the body. Maintain high blood pressure.
ZINC	Oysters, meats, liver, wheatgerm, pumpkin seeds, sunflower seeds.	Relieve angina and cirrhosis of the liver.	Important for normal growth, foetal growth, reproductive development, and the healing of wounds.

DEFICIENCIES

Lack of adequate vitamins and minerals can cause potentially serious diseases. But a varied diet with plenty of fruit and vegetables should provide the nutrition you require.

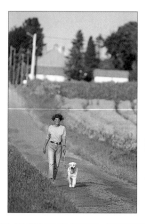

THE 'SUNSHINE VITAMIN'
Sunshine is an important source of vitamin D. It is created when ultraviolet light in sunlight acts on a substance in the skin. People who remain indoors all day may become deficient in vitamin D, which can cause softened bones.

In 1746, the naval doctor James Lind proved that eating a lemon a day stopped his sailors developing scurvy, the potentially fatal disease that weakens the body's connective tissue. However, it took another 170 years before scientists isolated its cause – vitamin C deficiency. This important discovery soon led to uncovering the causes of other deficiency diseases, including complete loss of eyesight (lack of vitamin A); beriberi, which is characterised by partial paralysis (lack of vitamin B_1); pellagra, which results in dermatitis, diarrhoea, and dementia (lack of vitamin B_3); and rickets, a disease in which the bones do not harden properly and become distorted (lack of vitamin D). These diseases are now rare in the West, but the health of a fifth of the global population is damaged through a lack of adequate vitamins and minerals.

If you eat a varied diet that includes fish and plenty of fruits and vegetables, you will probably get all the vitamins and minerals you need from your food. Certain groups of people, however, are still vulnerable to deficiencies. Vegans and vegetarians who do not eat eggs or meat may not get enough B_{12}, causing new red blood cells to develop abnormally, without sufficient haemoglobin, which is necessary for carrying oxygen around the body. This condition is known as megaloblastic anaemia. B_{12} deficiency can also arise due to poor absorption and this condition is known as pernicious anaemia. In spite of an increasing loss of sensation in the hands and feet, pernicious anaemia may go unnoticed until serious damage to the nervous system has already occurred.

People who stay indoors all day, such as institutionalised and very elderly people, may not get enough vitamin D. This may cause rickets in children and osteomalacia (softening of the bones) in adults.

Recommended dietary allowance

Different countries have established different daily levels or recommended daily allowances (RDAs) of each vitamin and mineral needed to prevent deficiency (see pp. 62 and 63). Levels in the United States are higher than they are in the United Kingdom, for instance, with a wider margin of nutritional safety. But RDAs can vary from your optimum requirements.

Many nutritionists are concerned that people do not eat a varied diet rich in fruits and vegetables (five servings per day) but instead one that contains too many snacks

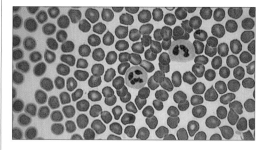

HEALTHY RED BLOOD CELLS
Red blood cells depend on iron, vitamin B_{12} and folic acid to form haemoglobin, which transports oxygen to, and carbon dioxide from, the body's cells.

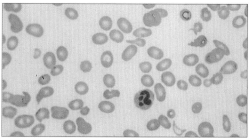

'SICK' RED BLOOD CELLS
A deficiency in vitamin B_{12} and folic acid can cause blood cells that lack haemoglobin and have less capacity for carrying oxygen; this gives rise to anaemia.

and fast foods. As a result, they believe that there is widespread inadequate nutrition – that many people have low or borderline levels of essential vitamins and minerals. Nutritionists are particularly worried about the levels of a range of minerals, including iron, calcium, zinc, magnesium, chromium and selenium and the vitamins A, C and E.

IRON

Iron in red blood cells is efficiently recycled and only a tiny amount is lost each day through faeces, urine and cells sloughed from the stomach. But, even though iron is stored by the body, iron deficiency is the most common mineral deficiency world-wide. It occurs when the body does not get enough iron over a long period of time and is unable to make sufficient haemoglobin which leads to anaemia.

In Western industrialised countries alone, it is estimated that as many as 20 to 30 per cent of women of child-bearing age do not possess adequate iron reserves. In the United Kingdom, 5 per cent of women in this age group are anaemic, while another 15 per cent have inadequate reserves of iron. Inadequate intake, poor absorption and blood loss through menstruation are the primary reasons for iron deficiency. Common symptoms are weakness, fatigue and shortness of breath. According to the

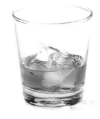

NUTRIENT DEPLETERS
Alcohol and some medications, such as antihistamines, diminish the beneficial effects of vitamin A.

CAUSES OF NUTRIENT DEPLETION

Vitamin loss occurs when foods are exposed to light and heat or cooked in large amounts of water. After foods are eaten, the effects of their vitamins and minerals in the body diminishes if certain other substances are consumed.

NUTRIENT	BEFORE EATING	AFTER EATING
A	Light, high temperatures, air, iron or copper kitchen utensils.	An excess of alcohol, smoking, antihistamines, antacids.
B_1	Baking powder, sulphur dioxide (preservative), leaching into cooking water, water loss during thawing.	An excess of alcohol.
B_2	Light, heat, alkaline conditions (baking with bicarbonate of soda), leaching into cooking water.	
B_3	Leaching into cooking water, water loss during thawing.	Isoniazid (antituberculosis drug).
B_6		Excessive protein foods.
B_{12}	Alkaline conditions (boiling in bicarbonate of soda).	An excess of alcohol, smoking.
FOLIC ACID	Processing at very high temperatures, light, leaching into cooking water.	An excess of alcohol.
C	Light, baking, air, alkaline conditions, iron or copper kitchen utensils, leaching into water when soaked.	Smoking.
D	Processing, freezing.	Barbiturates, laxatives, diuretics, anticonvulsive drugs.
E		Polyunsaturated fats.
K		Antibiotics, laxatives, diuretics.
CALCIUM AND ZINC	Not all minerals are destroyed by cooking or food preparation, but some leach into the cooking medium.	Smoking and caffeine affect calcium. Alcohol, caffeine and oestrogen affect zinc.

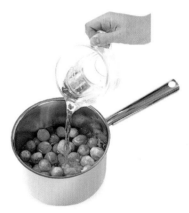

REDUCING LOSS OF NUTRIENTS
Boil vegetables in the minimum amount of water. Keep cooking time as short as possible.

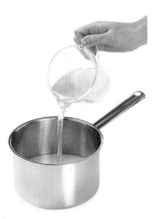

RECYCLING VITAMINS
Use the water that the vegetables were cooked in to make soups, sauces or gravies.

World Health Organization, about 700 million people worldwide have some degree of iron deficiency anaemia. Men and post-menopausal women usually have enough iron – their bodies store and recycle it efficiently. But the iron requirements of other groups may not be met sufficiently.

Women need extra iron during their fertile years. Menstruating women require more because of the regular monthly blood loss. Pregnant women need more iron because of increased blood volume and the requirements of the placenta and the developing foetus.

Infants, children and teenagers need more iron because of their rapid growth. Some studies have found that even minor iron deficiency may affect nonverbal learning and problem-solving capacity in children.

Dieters, especially women of child-bearing age, who eat only low-calorie meals are invariably getting an inadequate supply of iron. The less food they eat, the less likely they are to take in enough iron and other nutrients to meet the body's needs.

Vegetarians, especially young vegetarian women, and people who eat little red meat should eat alternative iron-rich foods such as apricots and fortified breakfast cereals.

Getting enough iron
There are two forms of dietary iron: haem, which is derived from meat and meat products, and non-haem, which comes from vegetable sources. Iron absorption varies according to its source, with haem iron having a better rate of absorption than non-haem iron. On average, 25 per cent of haem iron is absorbed no matter how much or how little your body needs. You can encourage a greater rate of absorption of both forms of iron by eating them with foods that are rich in vitamin C – cantaloupe, tomatoes or cabbage. Foods that are calcium-rich, however, can inhibit the body's ability to absorb iron. The cooking method you choose can affect the iron content of the food. The haem iron in meat, for example, can be degraded and converted to non-haem iron if the meat is cooked for a long time at a very high temperature.

CALCIUM
The bones act as a dynamic calcium storehouse for the rest of the body. Although they look inert, bones are continually losing and regaining calcium according to the body's needs. Hormones help to keep the calcium levels in the blood and other body fluids at a constant level, depositing any excess in the bones or removing them if they are needed elsewhere.

Peak bone mass
During growth, the skeleton increases in size, making extra demands on the body's calcium level. After growth stops, at about age 21 in boys and 18 in girls, the bone mass – the amount of bone and its calcium content together – continues to increase. At about age 30, what doctors term 'peak bone mass' is achieved. (This depends on the degree the diet provided calcium and other related nutrients, such as vitamin D, zinc, copper and manganese.) After this time, bone mass starts to decline very gradually because more bone is utilised by the body than is formed.

Because of hormonal changes, peak bone mass declines in a more pronounced manner in postmenopausal women. The decline in bone mass is normally not a problem for people whose calcium stores are adequate, but for those whose calcium intake was inadequate during the first three decades of life, the peak bone mass will not be enough to tolerate the gradual loss of bone mass over the years and a deficiency condition, osteoporosis, will result (see opposite).

Getting enough calcium
An inadequate calcium supply can occur if too little is consumed and absorbed or if too much is lost. Individuals at risk include growing infants, children and adolescents; pregnant women, who lose it to the foetus; and nursing mothers, whose calcium-rich milk goes to the infant.

The groups most at risk of calcium deficiency are women and adolescent girls; postmenopausal women (half of whom suffer from loss of bone density); and people who consume excessive amounts of tobacco and alcohol.

The United States has set a recommended daily allowance (RDA) of 1200 milligrams of calcium for people between the ages of 11 and 25 in an attempt to combat bone weakening. This daily allowance is high because this age group has the most efficient calcium absorption and can store the calcium for later years.

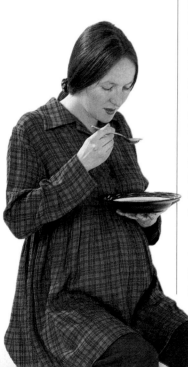

PREGNANCY
Lack of folic acid is linked with an increased risk of having a baby with such defects as spina bifida. Pregnant women, therefore, need to eat more foods that contain folic acid, such as spinach. Moreover, women who are hoping to become pregnant are advised to take supplements because the defect occurs in the 26th to 28th day of development, before most women know they are pregnant.

VITAMIN AND MINERAL SUPPLEMENTS

A huge profit is made by the companies who market vitamin and mineral supplements – about one in three adults takes them regularly. However, it is still not known how much good such supplements do for people who ordinarily are in good health.

A balanced diet with plenty of fresh fruit and vegetables will probably supply you with all the vitamins and minerals that you need. But produce in shops may not be fresh and certain vitamins, most notably C, degrade very quickly. The vitamin C content of apples, broccoli and strawberries, for instance, has been found to vary widely.

The time taken to transport fruits and vegetables to the shops and markets, the length of storage and whether or not the produce is seasonal will greatly affect its nutritional value. And, after preparation and cooking, the retention of many vitamins in such foods can be as little as 40 per cent of the original values.

In addition, many people eat unwisely and most have days when there is only time for snacks. Moreover, certain groups of people have higher than average nutritional requirements – people who are ill, the elderly, heavy drinkers and smokers, strict vegetarians and vegans, crash dieters and fussy eaters, athletes, children and pregnant and breastfeeding women. For those people who have inadequate dietary intakes, a nutritional boost provided by fortified meal replacements, such as breakfast cereals or a supplement, may be worthwhile.

Overdosing on supplements

Many people consume large quantities of certain supplements, especially vitamin C and iron, in the belief that a high amount

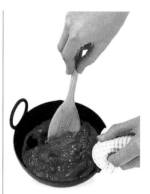

COOKING TO ADD IRON
You can improve the iron content of certain foods by cooking them in an iron pan or pot. Acidic foods, such as tomatoes, leach iron from the pan, which then becomes available as dietary iron.

THE EFFECTS OF OSTEOPOROSIS

Calcium is essential for bone health, since without it, bones become brittle and weak and prone to fracture. This condition is called osteoporosis and it affects women much more than men.

The hormone oestrogen is vital for the metabolism of calcium, especially in women. A woman's main source of oestrogen is her ovaries, but after the menopause, production stops. This means that calcium is incorporated into bone less efficiently and is also lost at a faster rate. The result is bones that become progressively weaker. Osteoporosis becomes even more likely if a woman had poor bone density early in life, smokes, or eats a low-calcium diet.

Many gynaecologists recommend hormone replacement therapy (HRT) for women who are at risk of osteoporosis as well as eating calcium-rich foods such as dark leafy greens and yoghurt. The National Osteoporosis Society of Great Britain recommends that women over 40 who are not on HRT should take the equivalent of 1500 mg of calcium a day and that women over 40 on HRT should take at least 1000 mg. Small amounts of zinc, copper and manganese enhance the absorption of calcium.

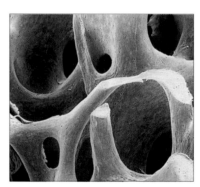

HEALTHY BONE
Calcium-rich bone maintains a resilient internal structure. This keeps it resistant to fracture. Eating foods that are rich in calcium and regular weight-bearing exercise help to keep bones strong.

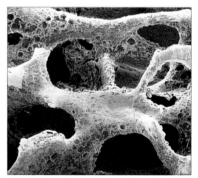

OSTEOPOROTIC BONE
Bone tissue affected by osteoporosis is much less dense, more brittle and prone to fracture. Your diet and the amount of weight-bearing exercise you took in your twenties and early thirties influences your chance of developing the condition.

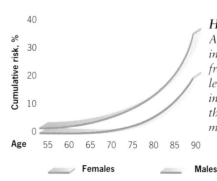

HIP FRACTURE RISKS
After the age of 50, there is an increasing risk of osteoporotic hip fracture. Naturally occurring low levels of oestrogen, combined with insufficient calcium intake, make the possibility of bone fractures more likely.

A vegetarian diet and pregnancy

Because of increased nutrient needs during pregnancy, vegetarian women are usually advised by doctors to supplement their diets with vitamin B$_{12}$, iron and calcium. But this does not mean relying on pills alone. Women should take care to augment their intakes of foods rich in these nutrients.

To obtain sufficient vitamin B$_{12}$, vegetarians should make sure that their diet contains eggs and milk. Vegans, on the other hand, will need to consume foods such as yeast extract and soya milks that are fortified with B$_{12}$.

A vegetarian and vegan diet rich in wholemeal bread, dark green vegetables and lentils will provide a good intake of iron, but this mineral can also be found in meat substitutes where it has been added by law. Combine iron-rich vegetarian foods with vitamin C to aid iron absorption.

Milk, cheese and yoghurt provide calcium, and vegetarians who include these foods in their diets will have adequate intakes. Vegans may suffer from low intakes and should eat ample dark green vegetables, pulses and tofu. They can also have white bread which, in the United Kingdom, is supplemented with calcium carbonate (chalk).

will increase the beneficial effects. However, megadoses – an amount that is ten times or more than the RDA – can be harmful.

The vitamins A, D and E are stored in the liver and, being fat soluble, can build up in the body. If taken regularly, doses of A and D that are five to ten times higher than the RDA can be toxic. People have become very ill as a result of eating large quantities of animal liver, which contains a great deal of vitamin A. Fish liver oil is a rich source of both A and D, but if you have too much, the oil is likely to make you vomit.

There does not appear to be any danger from a prolonged high intake of beta carotene. The only side effect is a yellowing of the skin, particularly the palms of the hands and soles of the feet.

Vitamin E, on the other hand, is not toxic in high doses. One hundred milligrams of vitamin E appears beneficial in thwarting heart disease, but some people take larger doses because they believe it prolongs life. However, an increased intake of something that does you good in nominal doses may not increase the benefits you receive.

SYMPTOMS OF NUTRIENT DEFICIENCY

Everybody needs a balanced intake of vitamins and minerals. But some people require a greater intake to meet particular needs. If they do not get an adequate supply, they may suffer problems that are signs of the nutrient deficiency.

NUTRIENT	DEFICIENCY SYMPTOMS	THOSE MOST AT RISK
A	Dry eyes, night blindness, poor growth and development, hardening of skin, impaired immunity.	Toddlers.
B$_1$	Fatigue, muscle weakness and nausea. Can lead to fatal illness called beriberi with heart failure.	Alcoholics, people on a staple diet of polished rice.
B$_2$	Dry and cracked skin, bloodshot eyes, sore lips and tongue.	People who do not drink milk.
B$_3$	Depression and tiredness. Severe deficiency leads to pellagra, which is characterised by dermatitis, diarrhoea and dementia.	People on a corn-based diet.
B$_6$	Convulsions.	Naturally occurring deficiency unknown.
B$_{12}$	Megaloblastic anaemia (abnormal red blood cells). Degeneration of the spinal cord, which leads to paralysis and death. May also cause mental confusion in the elderly.	Vegans, vegetarians, heavy drinkers, pregnant and lactating women. Deficiency can also be caused by malabsorption rather than dietary lack.
C	Slow wound healing, loose teeth, bleeding gums, easy bruising, recurrent infections, internal haemorrhaging, scurvy.	Smokers, the elderly.
D	Rickets (bones do not harden and become distorted in children), osteomalacia (softening of the bones in adults).	Children, the elderly, the housebound, individuals consuming a diet rich in unleavened bread (pitta) and brown rice.
E	Haemolytic anaemia, nerve damage.	Individuals with a diet high in polyunsaturated fats, especially fish oils.
CALCIUM	Rickets, osteomalacia.	Children, adolescents, pregnant and lactating women, vegans, the elderly.
IRON	Iron-deficiency anaemia – fatigue, shortness of breath.	Women who have heavy periods, pregnant women, vegetarians, sick or elderly people.

A regular intake of vitamin C and the B family, which are water-soluble, is necessary because they are not stored in the body and any excess is excreted in urine. This makes them mostly harmless in excess except for vitamins B_3 and B_6 and folic acid. Megadoses of B_3 can cause nausea, flushing and low blood pressure, and too much B_6, which some women take for premenstrual syndrome, can lead to irreversible nerve damage. Doses exceeding 25 milligrams per day should be avoided. Sudden high doses of vitamin C, however, may cause gastric disturbance.

Ideally, you should take supplements only on the recommendation of your doctor. Tests can establish whether or not a supplement is needed, especially when you are thinking of taking iron, selenium or zinc. Each can build up in toxic amounts that may damage body organs, including the liver, pancreas and heart.

No mineral should be routinely consumed in doses greater than ten times the RDA and even that practice should be short term.

Can vitamins treat disease?

The most publicised claims for the use of a vitamin in the treatment of disease were those put forward by the American scientist Linus Pauling (1901–94). Initially, he advocated the use of gram doses of vitamin C to ward off and treat colds, but later he went still further, suggesting that vitamin C could prevent all manner of human diseases, including cancer.

Pauling's unorthodox methods and sweeping claims eventually earned him the suspicion of the medical and scientific communities. Many studies were conducted to test his idea that vitamin C was a cold curative, but most of them indicate only small positive effects in reducing the incidence,

continued on page 74

TREATING DISEASE

In some cases, vitamin and mineral supplements move out of the realm of preventive medicine and into that of treatment. Doctors have discovered that many diseases and conditions can be relieved with proper supplementation. All these applications should be under the supervision of a doctor or clinical nutritionist.

▶ *Fat-soluble vitamins A, D, E and K can help people with cystic fibrosis, pancreatic diseases and malabsorption problems.*

▶ *Vitamin B_{12} (by injection) aids people who have had an operation on the stomach or small intestine. It is also given to people who have difficulty in absorbing vitamin B_{12}.*

▶ *Vitamin B_3 (niacin) lowers blood cholesterol.*

▶ *Vitamin B_6 eases premenstrual tension.*

▶ *B vitamins are recommended for individuals who are alcoholics. B vitamins help to heal damage to the body caused by excess alcohol consumption.*

▶ *Chromium helps to correct glucose intolerance.*

PREVENTING DISEASE WITH FOOD

Evidence from more than 300 studies has suggested that people who eat large quantities of the foods containing antioxidants – vitamins E, C and beta carotene – have a reduced risk of many cancers, heart disease, cataracts and stroke. Vitamin D also has disease-preventing properties, helping to stave off osteoporosis. It is the food itself that is particularly valuable, not the isolated nutrient that is found in supplements. Fruits and vegetables contain natural substances that enhance the absorption of vitamin C and have other protective properties.

SOURCES OF BETA CAROTENE
Orange, red and yellow vegetables and fruits are high in beta carotene and other carotenes that may help to reduce the risk of lung cancer. The fibre in these foods may contribute to a reduced risk of colon cancer.

SOURCES OF VITAMINS D AND E
Oily fish and fortified cereals are a good source of vitamin D, which helps to strengthen bones. Vegetable oils, sunflower seeds and nuts are rich in vitamin E and will help to prevent damage to fatty acids in the body.

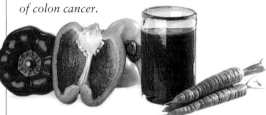

SOURCES OF VITAMIN C
Citrus fruits, broccoli and potatoes are rich in vitamin C, which is an effective cancer preventer and helps to block the formation of cancer-causing nitrosamines.

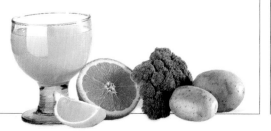

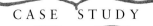
A Perimenopausal Woman

The time leading up to the menopause can be very challenging – the body you thought you knew undergoes a major internal transformation. As hormones ebb and flow, emotional changes, like moodiness and irritability, and physical ones, such as hot flushes and joint pain, may arise. You can help to counteract these effects by making positive changes in your diet, exercise patterns and attitude.

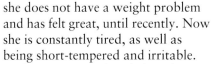

Ellen is a single 47-year-old executive. She recently left her job in a public relations firm to start her own business. Since then she has done hardly anything else but work. She has stopped seeing friends and exercising and no longer pays much attention to what she eats.

She starts her day with four cups of coffee, then snacks on biscuits, chocolate, crisps and similar food until dinner. Then she usually grabs a bowl of pasta, and washes it down with a glass or two of wine to help her to unwind. Despite her poor eating habits and lack of exercise, she does not have a weight problem and has felt great, until recently. Now she is constantly tired, as well as being short-tempered and irritable.

Ellen's menstrual cycle has also become irregular. In addition, she is sweating a lot. At first, she broke out into a sweat every afternoon, but now it happens twice a day. She feels frustrated by her lack of control over her own body and blames the stress of her business for her symptoms.

Frightened by her feelings of powerlessness, Ellen took a two-week holiday. As she unwound from the pressures of her job, she thought about what was happening to her. Could it be the menopause? She is sure this happens later and thinks her symptoms are simply stress-related.

Back at work, she has resumed her usual frenetic pace but finds that her symptoms have escalated. To keep her energy level up, she drinks more coffee and eats more sugary snacks. At night, to unwind, she drinks an extra glass of wine. But she finds that no matter how much sugar and caffeine she consumes, she still lacks energy. In addition, her nightly drinks no longer relax her. Ellen decides she needs to get help.

DIET
Sufficient calcium intake is essential as a woman ages to replace that being lost from the body. Eating a balanced diet (see p. 18) will also improve her mood and attitude, as well as relieve many menopausal symptoms.

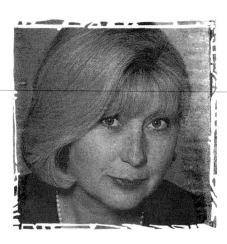

HEALTH
Physical symptoms such as hot flushes, night sweats, aches in the joints and stress incontinence are a few of the conditions associated with the onset of the menopause. Hot flushes can last for just a few seconds or up to several minutes.

FITNESS
A lack of exercise can exacerbate the emotional symptoms of the menopause, such as anxiety and depression. Inactivity can also increase the risks of osteoporosis and heart disease.

EATING HABITS
A busy and active life tends to leave little time for specially prepared and relaxing meals. Taking time to prepare meals will relieve tension.

EMOTIONAL HEALTH
Around the time of the menopause women may experience disconcerting mood swings. Anxiety and tearfulness can arise with only slight provocation and be followed by sudden, inexplicable euphoria.

WHAT SHOULD ELLEN DO?

Rather than reaching for coffee, sugar and alcohol, Ellen needs to take an honest look at what is going on in her life. Although her stress level has not really changed much, she seems less able to cope with it.

Ellen should make an appointment with her general practitioner or gynaecologist to find out whether she is undergoing the menopause. The menopause has a number of serious health implications – notably the increased risks of osteoporosis (see p. 69) and heart disease.

To find out more about what is happening to her body, Ellen should read more about female health. There are many books about women's health and the menopause in bookshops, and her local public library may also have a selection of relevant literature. Ellen could also talk to friends who have already experienced the menopause.

In addition, Ellen could become more familiar with the different therapies that may help to relieve menopausal symptoms. Hormone replacement therapy (HRT) works well to relieve hot flushes and night sweats and helps to avert osteoporosis and heart disease.

Relaxation therapies such as meditation can also offer relief as they calm the mind and body.

All this information will help to make Ellen feel more in control of what is going on in her body.

Action Plan

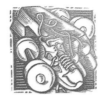

DIET
Find out about the diet recommended for women going through the menopause. (High-calcium foods, such as dairy products, are important for staving off osteoporosis.) Ellen also needs a good intake of vitamin D to aid the absorption and metabolism of calcium. Caffeine is a calcium depleter.

FITNESS
Plan to exercise regularly – at least three times a week. Brisk walking, aerobics and walking on a treadmill help to strengthen bone mass, which reduces the risk of osteoporosis. Decide whether to take up a sport or join a fitness club.

HEALTH
Arrange to see a doctor. (May need various health checks – breast and pelvic examinations, including a mammogram and cervical smear – as well as height, weight, blood pressure and cholesterol.) Have hormone levels measured through a blood test). Self-examine breasts once a month.

EMOTIONAL HEALTH
Contact a local self-help group. Learn to anticipate mood swings and investigate various natural and medical remedies. For example, certain herbal preparations are said to be calming. HRT is effective for emotional symptoms and helps to increase energy levels.

EATING HABITS
Take time to prepare meals. If too busy or tired during the week, make more time-consuming, nourishing meals at the weekend and freeze uneaten food in portion-size containers. Reheat the food after work or the gym. Stop snacking on chocolates and biscuits. Try eating smaller meals frequently.

HOW THINGS TURNED OUT FOR ELLEN

Ellen's gynaecologist tells her she is perimenopausal. This stage, which may last several years, precedes the last menstrual period. Hormone levels begin to drop and, during this time, many physical symptoms of the menopause, such as frequent hot flushes and night sweats, are experienced. Ellen's doctor recommends a nutritionist, who provides a diet to help Ellen's body to cope with its changes. This new diet consists of four well-balanced low-fat, high-fibre meals a day. She has to eat plenty of whole grains, fresh fruits and vegetables and small amounts of fish and lean meats.

Ellen now drinks only one cup of coffee a day and has cut down on fast food. She also drinks more water to replace the amount she loses through sweating. For snacks, she eats calcium-rich foods like low-fat milk, yoghurt and cheese.

Eating regular nutritious meals gives her more energy and reduces her moodiness and irritability.

In the evening, Ellen stops work an hour early and walks part of the way home. She has joined a health club with a friend and several days a week she spends some time exercising there or at home. She has become better at unwinding and the combination of exercise and relaxation is invigorating.

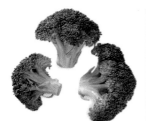

VITAMIN C
Just 100 g (3½ oz) of cooked broccoli supplies the recommended daily allowance for vitamin C.

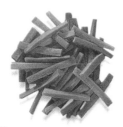

BETA CAROTENE
Eating a 100 g (3½ oz) carrot meets the daily need for beta carotene.

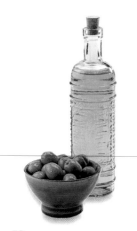

VITAMIN E
Vegetable oils are a good source of vitamin E. Use unsaturated oils, for example olive, when cooking instead of the more harmful saturated fats, such as butter.

easing the symptoms and shortening the duration of the common cold. Even these effects may be due to vitamin C's antioxidant properties and its enhancement of immune functions.

Recently, however, interest in vitamin C as a possible means of preventing colds has led to more research, and some of Pauling's initial observations are stimulating further investigation as a result.

FREE RADICALS AND ANTIOXIDANTS

Current research has uncovered so-called unstable molecules (free radicals), which may be causal factors in a number of degenerative diseases, including cancer and heart disease. This theory has led to further investigations to clarify the relationship between free radical molecules and antioxidants, such as beta carotene, which mop them up and may therefore reduce the risk of these diseases. Several studies suggest that vitamin A and possibly the other carotenes may help to prevent breast cancer.

The evidence that vitamin E reduces the incidence of heart disease is even stronger. One study tested 16 000 men between 40 and 59 years of age from 16 different places in Europe. The higher the level of vitamin E in their blood, the lower their death rates from heart disease. Similar associations have been observed for vitamin C and beta carotene. All are antioxidants, and it appears that they function as a protective 'brigade' with vitamin C as the first line of defence, vitamin E and other compounds in the middle, and beta carotene as a last line of defence against free radicals.

However, these findings do not mean that you should start taking supplements of these antioxidants. Although the effects of vitamin supplements are still being debated, there is no argument that eating more fruit, vegetables and grains that are rich in antioxidants is beneficial. It is therefore advisable to make sure you follow the current dietary recommendations for these foods. To ensure an adequate intake of vitamins, minerals and other nutrients, health experts recommend that you consume a certain number of food portions each day: six to eleven servings of cereals and potatoes; five servings of fruits and vegetables; two to three servings of dairy products, preferably low-fat; two to three servings of protein foods, such as meat, seafood, pulses and eggs; and only a very small amount of fat.

ALUMINIUM AND ALZHEIMER'S DISEASE

Alzheimer's disease is a condition – to date irreversible – in which the brain's nerve cells progressively degenerate and cause the brain to shrink. In different studies, scientists have found high levels of aluminium in the brain of some Alzheimer's patients and a concentration of cases in areas with high levels of aluminium in the drinking water.

But controversy rages about whether excessive aluminium is the cause, or a result, of the neurological damage in Alzheimer's disease. Scientists are not sure that changes in the brain and other body organs are caused by the disease. Alzheimer's might ease the entry of aluminium and other metals to the brain.

However, in the wake of the evidence linking Alzheimer's and aluminium, many people have become concerned with the safety of aluminium cooking utensils. But even if the metal does leach into food,

scientists are not sure if dietary aluminium can be absorbed through the intestines. It is now thought that drinking plenty of fluids and eating a balanced diet may be of more practical benefit in warding off Alzheimer's disease than attempting to be sure that no aluminium enters your diet through cooking utensils. You can, however, choose from a wide range of pots and pans made in other materials, particularly stainless steel and ceramics.

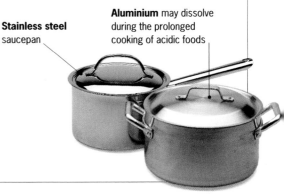

Stainless steel saucepan

Aluminium may dissolve during the prolonged cooking of acidic foods

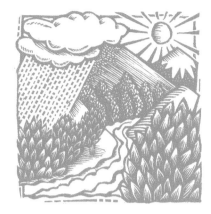

CHAPTER 6

THE FLUID FACTOR

---

*What you drink, when you drink and how
much you drink is as important to a healthy diet
as the food you eat. All living cells and organs need
water to function. Water is the basis of essential
body fluids such as blood and lymph; it lubricates
joints; it is needed to form the basis of saliva;
it provides a protective cushion for the body's tissues
and it helps to eliminate digestive waste from the
body. Water, skimmed milk and unsweetened fruit
juices are the most beneficial fluids, while alcoholic
and caffeinated drinks – tea, coffee and certain
colas – may be harmful if taken in excess.*

ARE YOU DRINKING ENOUGH WATER?

You can live for several weeks without food, but without water you will die in just a few days. Luckily, most people have a ready source, although there may be doubts about its quality.

THE RIGHT AMOUNT

As a rough guide, the World Health Organisation recommends that everyone drink eight glasses of water a day. Drink more water if

▶ *You take part in strenuous exercise.*

▶ *The weather is hot.*

▶ *You are at a high altitude.*

▶ *You are ill, especially with diarrhoea or fever.*

▶ *You are menopausal and suffering from hot flushes and night sweats.*

In 1987, Greece experienced a ten-day heatwave with temperatures reaching 43°C (110°F). More than 1000 people died, most of them elderly, mainly from the effects of dehydration – loss of fluids and body salt. This is an extreme example of what can happen if the body is not kept properly hydrated. Clearly, the high temperature was the major factor contributing to the tragedy, but even in lower temperatures, it is important to drink enough water to replace the amount lost through bodily functions – breathing, perspiration, urination and defecation.

On average, you lose 1 to 2 litres (1¾–3½ pints) of water a day, and the rate is significantly increased, perhaps up to 5 litres (8¾ pints), through perspiration during periods of physical exertion or in areas of very hot climate and high altitude. As long as the lost fluid is replenished, there is no problem. But other factors, such as your state of health, can lead to a dangerous increase in water loss. Fever, vomiting, diarrhoea and blood loss all cause dehydration. The treatment for these illnesses includes the controlled replacement of lost water.

AN ADEQUATE SUPPLY

If the body does not take in enough water, those functions requiring the action of water, such as the dilution and evacuation of toxins, lead to water being drawn from the cells to make up the balance. This results in dehydration of the cells, which shrivel and cease to function properly. The body reacts swiftly to water loss: losing just 1 per cent is enough to make you thirsty, while extreme rates of dehydration can lead to heat stroke and may even be fatal.

SUFFERING FROM THE EFFECTS OF HEAT

Insufficient water intake is one of the main causes of heat exhaustion – signalled by cramps, nausea and headache. Sufferers will also have shallow breathing and clammy skin. If heat exhaustion is not treated, heat stroke may develop: sweating stops, the skin becomes flushed and there may be loss of consciousness, coma and death. Individuals suffering from heat exhaustion should lie in a cool place and sip an oral rehydration solution – 1 teaspoon of salt, 8 teaspoons of sugar in 1 litre (1¾ pints) of water, see p. 155. If an individual loses consciousness, place him or her in the recovery position until consciousness is regained. Then administer the rehydration solution. Seek medical help immediately.

HEAT EXHAUSTION
A sufferer will feel nauseated and sweat profusely. The diagram below shows the response of skin to heat.

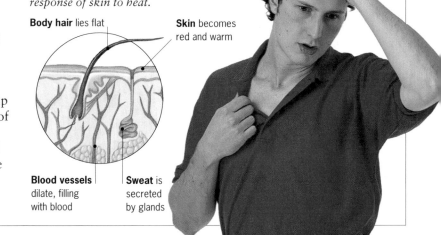

Body hair lies flat

Skin becomes red and warm

Blood vessels dilate, filling with blood

Sweat is secreted by glands

Dehydration becomes a major threat when 10 per cent of a person's weight is lost. For example, a 75 kilogram (165 pound) man would lose 7.5 kilograms (16.5 pounds).

The sensation of thirst is the body's way of saying that it needs more water. A dry mouth is the result of the blood becoming excessively salty and drawing moisture from the salivary glands to redress the balance. Usually a glass or two of water is enough to stop you feeling thirsty, but it may not be enough to prevent dehydration. Thirst is an imperfect warning system, however, because it is not triggered until dehydration has already begun. Therefore your thirst may tend to be quenched before you have drunk an adequate amount of water. So it is a good idea to drink enough water to satisfy your thirst and then drink some more – another glass or two. However, excessive thirst can also be a sign of diabetes mellitus.

Are you drinking the right water?

Water from the tap in most developed countries has for a long time been regarded as safe to drink. In recent years, however, many people have become concerned about pollutants seeping into the water supply, and the rising sales of filters and bottled water reflect this general unease.

Tap water comes from two main sources: surface water and ground water. Surface water includes lakes, reservoirs, rivers and streams, which supply most major cities, while ground water – a more common supply for rural areas – comes from underground sources such as cave complexes where water collects.

The treatment of water

With their several stages of filtration, aeration and disinfection, modern water-treatment systems are highly sophisticated, and, even internationally, most of the water supplied to the public is safe to drink. This is particularly true of urban areas where the consumer is served by municipal water systems. In rural areas, where the demand on small community systems is greater, and especially where water is drawn from private wells, extra vigilance is more important.

The risk of becoming ill as a result of consuming contaminated drinking water is very small. Most drinking water is safer now than ever before. This is borne out by the low incidence of disease caused by

WATERY FOODS

Half the water your body needs comes from foods. Vegetables and fruits contain more liquid than solid matter.

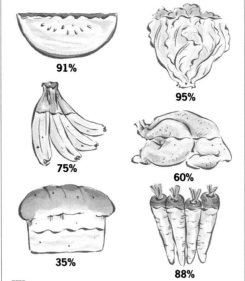

91%

95%

75%

60%

35%

88%

WATER LEVELS IN FOOD
Watermelons are almost entirely water, while the proportion of water in lettuce is 95 per cent, in carrots 88 per cent and in bananas about 75 per cent. Poultry is about 60 per cent water and water even goes to make up about 35 per cent of bread.

WHICH DRINK IS BEST?

Almost any fluid will do for replenishment, but water, pure and simple, is best. The next best are pure fruit juices and low-fat milk. Caffeinated and alcoholic drinks do not replace lost water because they act as diuretics, making the kidneys produce more urine than they would normally. Drinking sweet fizzy drinks increases the amount of sugar in your diet, which may cause tooth decay.

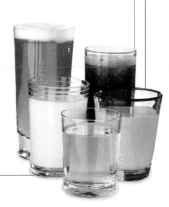

QUENCHING YOUR THIRST
Choose plain water, juice or low-fat milk instead of alcoholic, caffeinated or fizzy drinks.

Fluid intake and excercise

During periods of prolonged strenuous exercise, such as cycling or marathon running, it is particularly important to replenish the extra fluid that is lost. Many nutritionists recommend that endurance athletes take isotonic drinks to rehydrate the body. These commercial drinks contain small amounts of carbohydrate and sodium, and are absorbed by the body faster than water. The carbohydrate also supplies needed fuel.

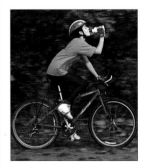

TOPPING UP YOUR FLUID INTAKE
While exercising, have an isotonic drink or a glass of water every 15 to 20 minutes.

Filtering water

Water filters are a cheap and popular way of cleaning water, but if misused they can cause more problems than they solve. They work by using layers of activated charcoal (charcoal that is honeycombed with tiny channels). As water passes through these channels, chemicals stick to the walls and are filtered out. But if the activated charcoal or carbon filters are not changed regularly, they can become a breeding ground for harmful bacteria. And although filters effectively remove cloudiness from the water and some metals, these filters are inadequate to remove viruses or harmful bacteria, and few cut down on the amount of inorganic chemicals such as lead and other heavy metals or nitrates.

contaminated water today compared to the time before chlorination and controls on water sources were imposed. But the amount of chemicals and metals being discharged into the environment by industrial plants and modern agricultural methods is putting a burden on water sources, and inevitably some pollution occurs. Unfortunately, the appearance, taste and smell of drinking water are not effective criteria for determining its quality. But in Britain you can be assured that the water reaching your home is safe to drink because water companies treat water to remove any potentially harmful substances and are required to conduct stringent tests in order to comply with British and European regulations. These controls are among the highest standards for drinking water in the world; every year the Drinking Water Inspectorate (an independent government watchdog) makes detailed checks on all UK water suppliers to see that they are meeting current standards.

If you are at all worried about the quality of your water supply you should contact your local water company; they will provide details on their water quality records or will visit your home and test your water supply.

In Britain, parents should not worry about giving tap water to babies or young children. Given the strict quality controls, it is probably safer than bottled water.

Organic pollutants

Contamination by organic chemicals is not new. Most of these chemicals are formed from decaying matter and therefore occur naturally. As well as these pollutants there may be traces of synthetic organic chemicals developed in industrial solvents, pesticides and herbicides. Whether natural or synthetic, organic chemicals are usually found only in very dilute amounts in drinking water, and these substances are reduced to levels which in practice cannot be detected. The UK government and the European Community have set standards for the levels of 57 substances found in drinking water and the water authorities test regularly for them.

Chlorination

Chlorine is used as a disinfectant to kill or inactivate any bacteria that may be present in water. Most of it is then removed except for a small amount, the 'residual chlorine', which is left to maintain the quality of the water supply during its journey through the system to your tap. The exact amount of residual chlorine found in your home supply varies, depending on factors such as the closeness of your home to the treatment works. Some people are more sensitive to the taste of chlorine than others, but you can get rid of the taste by letting the water stand for a while in the refrigerator.

POSSIBLE THREATS TO WATER SUPPLIES

A range of pollutants can enter a surface water supply through acid rain, pesticide run-off in rural areas, rainwater run-off in cities and industrial waste from manufacturing plants. Ground water supplies are exposed to a more limited range of pollutants, but generally in higher concentrations. Fertilisers may sink through the soil, and chemical wastes seep from poorly maintained underground fuel tanks, waste-storage sites or simply from carelessly discarded household products.

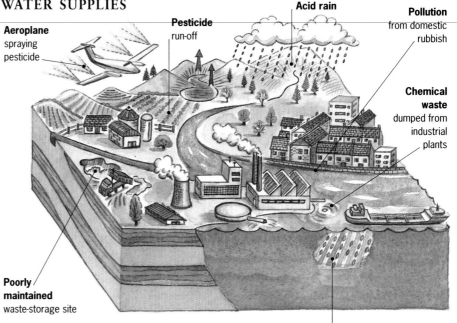

Aeroplane spraying pesticide

Pesticide run-off

Acid rain

Pollution from domestic rubbish

Chemical waste dumped from industrial plants

Poorly maintained waste-storage site

Outflow of oil from tanker

REDUCING LEAD

If you live in an area where the water is 'soft', you can reduce the danger from lead by following these simple steps.

▶ *Do not use hot water for drinking or cooking, since hot water dissolves more lead from pipes.*

▶ *Let your cold tap run for a while first thing in the morning; lead can build up overnight or in water that has sat in the pipe for a few hours. Flushing the toilet or running cold water in the shower will also help to wash the pipes of any accumulated levels of lead.*

▶ *Let water run for a few seconds before drinking from the cold tap during the day.*

Heavy metals

People living in a chalk or limestone area have 'hard' water, which contains calcium salts that make the water slightly alkaline. Those who live in a granite area have 'soft' water, which is fairly acidic. Lead, copper and cadmium seep into the water supply in areas where the water is soft, because soft water has a more corrosive effect on the metals used in water pipes than hard water.

Of all the heavy metals, the most dangerous is probably lead because of its high toxicity. Lead is not usually present in water sources but gets into drinking water because of the action of soft water on lead pipes, which were once used to connect properties to the water main, and for household plumbing. Lead has not been used for these purposes since the late 1970s, but some older properties still have lead pipework or copper pipes with lead solder. If you think your household is at risk you can ask your water company to test your pipes.

The question of fluoride

Fluoride is a vital micronutrient that occurs naturally in soils and rocks and may occur in drinking water. It is used to strengthen teeth (particularly children's) by forming mineral crystals in the tooth enamel. Fluoride both strengthens the enamel and prevents naturally occurring bacteria from causing decay. Most doctors believe that fluoride is quite safe, yet some claim that it can be dangerous. They point to a few studies that have linked it to the increased incidence of cancer and reduced thyroid activity. But the methodology of these studies has been questioned and most scientists discount them. Communities whose water is fluoridated have shown no increase in the incidence of cancer or any other of the alleged ill effects.

At one part per million parts of water – the standard level of fluoride used in water fluoridation – fluoride is perfectly safe and helps to reduce the risk of dental caries. The only adverse effect is found in regions with water supplies that have naturally occurring high levels of fluoride (about eight times the level used in artificially fluoridated supplies). In these areas there have been cases of dental fluorosis, a pitting and discoloration of the teeth. Children who still have their first set of teeth are particularly at risk from fluorosis, and should brush their teeth with toothpastes containing the lowest levels of fluoride. Most brands of toothpaste, however, are safe for the rest of the family.

IS MINERAL WATER HEALTHIER THAN TAP WATER?

Bottled mineral water, both still and sparkling, is one of the growth industries of the last decade. The minerals most often found in these waters are calcium, magnesium, potassium and sulphate. Many claims are made about the health benefits of mineral water, but although it may taste better, it is unlikely to have much effect on health one way or the other. In addition, the sudden boom in bottled water sales means that regulation has yet to keep pace fully, and both the levels of purity and the claims made about beneficial effects are open to doubt. The high mineral content of some waters makes them unsuitable for young children, while people with high blood pressure should avoid waters with a high sodium content. Always check the labels of the various brands.

While there is no hard evidence that mineral water provides greater safety than tap water, it can be a useful, if often expensive, alternative in the event of short-term pollution. In general, bottled water should be drunk in countries where the purity of the water supply is questionable – and in such places it should also be used for brushing your teeth. But where water conditions are deemed acceptable, bottled water may not actually provide any greater level of safety.

Rocketing sales

The amount of mineral water consumed has been rising for more than a decade. In the United Kingdom in 1980, only 30 million litres of mineral water were sold. By 1990 the figure had multiplied by 14. In the United States, sales have increased from 3582 million litres in 1982 to 8543 million litres in 1992. Whether for health, fashion or preference, the market is growing increasingly larger each year.

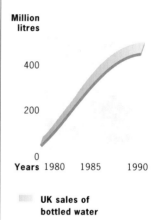

Million litres

400

200

0

Years 1980 1985 1990

▨ **UK sales of bottled water**

Drinking mineral water in restaurants

If you are concerned about the purity of water in a restaurant, order bottled water and make sure the bottle is opened in front of you. This way you will know that the original contents have not been replaced by water from the tap or from a soda siphon.

TO YOUR HEALTH

Research into an unexpectedly low rate of heart disease in France has pointed to health benefits from red wine, but in excess the bad effects of alcohol soon outweigh the good.

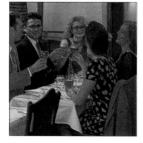

STAYING IN CONTROL Make sure you have something to eat before you have a drink and while you drink.

The French are justly famed for their food and their wines, so their high-cholesterol diet – pâté de foie gras, cassoulet, croissants – and their reputation as Europe's major smokers and wine drinkers, along with their lukewarm attitude towards exercise, would seem to be a recipe for rampant heart disease. Yet the incidence of heart disease in France is far lower than in the rest of Europe or America.

French adults drink an average of 2.5 glasses of red wine a day and often let their children drink watered-down wine at mealtimes. In recent years, some scientists have put forward the theory that this habit of drinking red wine may indeed help to prevent heart disease.

PROTECTING YOUR HEART

Alcohol raises the levels of protective substances in the blood called high-density lipoproteins (HDLs), which actively remove cholesterol. The less cholesterol there is in the blood, the less chance there is of the arteries clogging up with fatty deposits and bringing on a heart attack.

All alcohol, drunk in moderation, has this effect, but naturally occurring tannins and some of the other chemicals in red wine are thought to slow the oxidation of the HDLs, keeping them active longer.

A healthy amount

The operative term is 'moderation'. Experts emphasise that the window of opportunity for deriving positive effects from alcohol is quite narrow – up to three drinks a day for men and no more than two for women. A 'drink' here means 85 millilitres (3 fluid ounces) of wine. More than that and the bad effects start to outweigh the good.

Moderate consumption of red wine also seems to reduce the stickiness of blood platelets helping to prevent blood clots. As all alcohol produces this effect, people with bleeding conditions, such as haemophilia, should avoid drinking alcohol because it can bring on cerebral haemorrhaging.

Examples of one unit

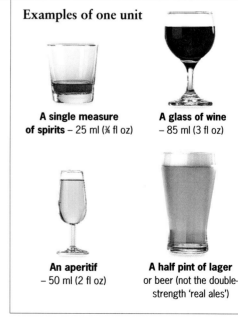

A single measure of spirits – 25 ml (¾ fl oz)

A glass of wine – 85 ml (3 fl oz)

An aperitif – 50 ml (2 fl oz)

A half pint of lager or beer (not the double-strength 'real ales')

Other beneficial effects of red wine

Recent research has shown that the body may need naturally occurring chemicals called antioxidants to stay healthy. Red wine contains polyphenols, potent sources of antioxidants. The value of antioxidants is that they neutralise free radicals. These are molecules that oxidise harmful substances in the body but that can also run amok, turning on the body's own cells. A surfeit of these free radicals is thought to contribute to many degenerative diseases – including heart disease and cancer – and even hasten the ageing process itself.

An unresolved debate

It has to be said, however, that the case for red wine is not entirely won. Although surveys point statistically to health benefits from drinking red wine, there is still the possibility that these benefits may have more to do with the character of red wine drinkers than with the wine itself. An ongoing study by Dr Arthur Klatsky and his colleagues at the Kaiser Permanente Medical Center, Oakland, California, has found that wine drinkers are more likely than beer drinkers to be moderate in their consumption, to smoke less or not at all and to be better educated about dietary matters.

Also, the Mediterranean way of drinking wine – in moderate quantities with meals consisting of the healthier diet of lean cuts of meat, fresh vegetables and olive oil – may go further towards solving what many nutritional scientists have called the French Paradox. And it may actually be the foods wine drinkers eat that help to provide protection against heart disease (see p. 114).

Although the potential health benefits of red wine may seem appealing, they are not a rationale for excessive drinking. Rates of liver cirrhosis and other alcohol-related diseases are actually much higher in France

---

THE PERILS OF EXCESSIVE DRINKING

As reports of the benefits of moderate drinking increase, many people may ignore the dangers of excessive alcohol consumption. Alcohol slows reaction time and disrupts orientation, so operating machinery, driving or crossing a road can be dangerous. But many people drink regularly without suffering too greatly from drunkenness and assume that their drinking is not harmful. If you regularly drink substantial amounts of alcohol, however, you may permanently damage your liver, heart and brain, and may be increasing your risk of falling prey to certain cancers. Such fatal conditions as cirrhosis of the liver are directly related to alcohol consumption. Aside from its devastating long-term effects, alcohol immediately begins to attack several of the body's systems and, although real damage requires persistent alcohol abuse, the effects of a hangover can be alarming.

THE BEST REMEDY
The first step after diagnosis of any alcohol-related health problem should be to stop drinking.

Depression
Heavy alcohol consumption gradually destroys the brain cells, and can result in depression, memory loss and intellectual deterioration

Liver disease
Persistent and excessive consumption may lead to fatty liver, alcoholic hepatitis, cirrhosis and liver cancer

Digestive disorders
Heavy drinkers may suffer from digestive tract diseases, such as gastritis, pancreatitis and cancer of the upper digestive tract

Nerve damage
Malnutrition, common among alcoholics, disturbs nerve functioning, causing symptoms such as cramps and numbness

Mouth and throat cancer
High levels of alcohol intake increase the risk of cancers of the mouth, tongue and throat

Heart disease
Heavy drinkers are more susceptible to coronary heart disease and hypertension (high blood pressure) and are more likely to suffer a stroke

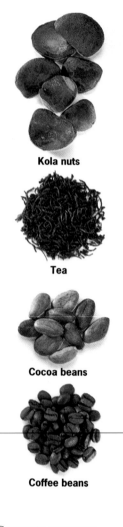

Kola nuts

Tea

Cocoa beans

Coffee beans

CAFFEINE SOURCES
Plant products contain-
ing caffeine, such as kola
nuts, tea, cocoa beans
and coffee beans, are
found all over the world.

than in Britain. And several studies have shown that habitual teetotalers, such as Seventh Day Adventists, live healthy lives.

WOMEN AND ALCOHOL

How much alcohol in the body may be considered safe depends on such things as weight, age, diet, genetics and illnesses suffered, but women in general should drink less alcohol than men. The reason is not just that women tend to have smaller frames proportionally, but also that their bodies contain more fat, in which alcohol will not dissolve. And, since women have less water in their bodies than men, their alcohol intakes do not become as diluted. Therefore, after a woman drinks the same amount of alcohol as a man, a higher concentration appears in her blood than in that of a man of the same weight. This makes women more prone to liver disease. Some research also suggests that an excessive consumption of alcohol increases the risk of breast cancer.

Drinking during pregnancy

Alcohol can cause foetal alcohol syndrome (FAS). FAS was first identified in the mid 1970s by researchers at the University of Washington, who studied birth defects and growth abnormalities among babies of women who drank heavily. FAS can lead to the baby being born with conditions such as a hare lip, cleft palate, flattened face, heart defects, deformed limbs and mental retardation. Such babies also tend to suffer growth retardation and poor muscle function.

Some researchers claim that as little as one drink a day during pregnancy can cause low birth-weight in babies; the equivalent of two glasses of wine per day can produce a one in ten chance of FAS.

Doctors advise women not to drink at all while they are trying to conceive or during the first 12 weeks of pregnancy. However, many doctors acknowledge that just a few glasses of wine taken before confirmation of pregnancy are unlikely to do harm.

THE HIGHS AND LOWS OF CAFFEINE

Caffeine has become an indispensable part of modern living. Almost everyone gets a lift from a morning cup of tea or coffee, and all age groups are avid consumers of caffeine, since in addition to coffee and tea it is present in colas and other soft drinks, cocoa and chocolate. (Also see page 100.)

The ability of caffeine to increase alertness and ward off sleep is well known. Long-distance lorry drivers, night workers, and students studying for exams welcome the lift that a cup of coffee brings. Not only does it prevent sleepiness, it actually helps the thought processes to become clearer, sharpens sensory perception and improves reaction time. After only two cups of coffee (or the equivalent) driving skills may improve. Caffeine also prevents lapses of concentration and reduces irritability. It is popular with dieters because it raises the basal metabolic rate (the rate at which heat is produced when the body is at rest), so that calories are burnt up more quickly.

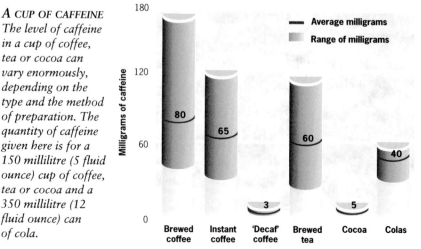

CAFFEINE LEVELS IN DIFFERENT DRINKS

A 150 millilitre (5 fluid ounce) cup of ground coffee contains about 80 milligrams of caffeine. The levels in other drinks, however, can be surprisingly high. An equal cup of brewed tea, for example, contains about 60 milligrams of caffeine. The 'strength' of coffee or tea is a good indication of the amount of caffeine. A strong tea, such as Assam, brewed for a long time contains more caffeine than weaker China or Ceylon.

A CUP OF CAFFEINE
The level of caffeine in a cup of coffee, tea or cocoa can vary enormously, depending on the type and the method of preparation. The quantity of caffeine given here is for a 150 millilitre (5 fluid ounce) cup of coffee, tea or cocoa and a 350 millilitre (12 fluid ounce) can of cola.

— Average milligrams

Range of milligrams

Milligrams of caffeine

180 — 120 — 60 — 0

Brewed coffee: 80
Instant coffee: 65
'Decaf' coffee: 3
Brewed tea: 60
Cocoa: 5
Colas: 40

Adverse effects

The bad news is that drinking cup after cup of coffee may be harmful to your health. Large doses of caffeine can make the heart beat faster and cause irregular beats. For this reason, caffeine has been linked to an increased risk of high blood pressure.

For dieters caffeine is a mixed blessing, since in addition to burning off calories, it also stimulates the release of insulin, which causes blood sugar to drop, creating feelings of hunger. So caffeine is only an aid to weight loss if the dieter is able to successfully ignore the hunger pangs that follow.

Too much coffee may result in tremors and inability to sleep. People who habitually drink up to 12 cups of strong coffee a day complain of symptoms ranging from sweating to anxiety. These symptoms disappear after just 36 hours without drinking coffee. People who suffer from gastric irritation or ulcers should avoid caffeine because it stimulates acid secretion in the stomach.

Children and caffeine

Growing children are also at risk from caffeine. Although they tend not to drink much tea or coffee, they do consume cola drinks that contain the drug. Because children are smaller than adults, they take in proportionally more caffeine from each cola drink and it therefore has a greater effect. One cola drink for a child may be the equivalent of four cups of coffee for an adult. Many countries now limit the caffeine level in cola drinks, but caffeine-free soft drinks may be better for children.

DECAFFEINATING COFFEE

Concern about the safety of chemicals used for decaffeinating coffee has led to the development of various water methods. For example, the Swiss water method retains most of the bean's taste by soaking beans in flavour-charged water. A more common water method is shown below.

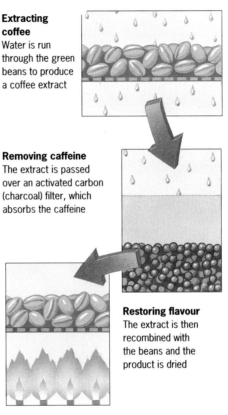

Extracting coffee
Water is run through the green beans to produce a coffee extract

Removing caffeine
The extract is passed over an activated carbon (charcoal) filter, which absorbs the caffeine

Restoring flavour
The extract is then recombined with the beans and the product is dried

---

HINTS ON CUTTING DOWN

You should limit your daily intake of caffeine to 200–250 milligrams or about three cups of brewed coffee. Gradually reducing your caffeine intake, rather than suddenly stopping, will help to prevent withdrawal symptoms such as headaches, lethargy and irritability.

▶ *If you normally drink coffee or tea from a mug, switch to a smaller cup.*

▶ *Change from ground coffee to instant.*

▶ *Drink decaffeinated coffee every other cup.*

▶ *Mix decaffeinated coffee with regular coffee to reduce total caffeine intake.*

▶ *Swap your strong tea for a weak one.*

▶ *Brew the tea for a shorter time than usual.*

▶ *Drink decaffeinated colas and other soft drinks.*

COFFEE SUBSTITUTES

When cutting down your caffeine intake be aware that you may be replacing your caffeine-rich drinks with something worse. Many soft drinks have high sugar levels, colourings and preservatives. But there are also dangers in drinking some herbal teas. A popular tea made from the roots of the kava plant is associated with hallucinations and dimmed vision. Another tea is made from the root bark of the sassafras tree, which has been linked with depression and hypothermia. Of course, most generally available herbal teas are harmless, and you can check more unusual ones with a herbalist.

HEALTHY BREW
Some herbal teas, such as rosehip, camomile, mint and vervain, are usually safe to drink in moderation. Alternatively, drink hot water flavoured with fresh lemon or lime. Fruit drinks that are brewed in hot water are also an enjoyable substitute for coffee.

Juicy goodness
Blend your own fruits and vegetables for delicious liquid refreshment and concentrated goodness.

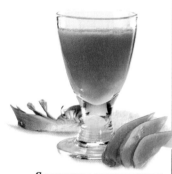

SOOTHING INDIGESTION
Papaya and pineapple juice may help to ease indigestion. The fruits' enzymes – papain in papaya and bromelin in pineapple – ease pain in the upper abdomen.

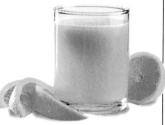

PREVENTING CANCER
A cocktail of red pepper and carrot is a rich source of the antioxidants beta carotene and vitamin C.

ABSORBING IRON
Fresh citrus juices make ideal accompaniments to meals. They contain plenty of vitamin C, which helps the body to absorb iron from foods.

THE JOYS OF JUICE

Fresh fruit and vegetable juice drinking has become much more widespread in recent years. Many people start each day with a glass of freshly squeezed orange juice, while others harvest their own crops of fruits and vegetables to press themselves, or follow diet regimes that are based on juices.

The health benefits

Most fresh fruits and vegetables are excellent sources of the antioxidant vitamins, beta carotene and vitamins C and E. These nutrients, research suggests, help to neutralise the harmful effects of the body's free radicals, which have been linked to ageing, heart disease and cancer (see p. 94).

Juices can also make you feel healthier because they contain plant enzymes that aid digestion. It is even claimed that juices are able to alleviate many common complaints such as sore throats and insomnia. But fruit juices such as apple and citrus juices naturally contain about 10 per cent sugar and, if consumed frequently throughout the day, will cause tooth decay.

Making your own

Although juices do not pack as much of a punch nutritionally as the raw, fibrous fruit or vegetable, they are often tastier. Carrot juice is a notable example.

Juices are also a good way to boost your vitamin intake. In most cases a glass of fresh juice provides several times the recommended levels of vitamins and minerals, and because they are water-based, the body will excrete any excess.

Freshly squeezed juices are better than the shop-bought variety because vitamin C diminishes with time and with exposure to air. They are also more likely to be free of any additives. Citrus fruits can be squeezed by hand, but with a juicing machine you can make a variety of cocktails. Thoroughly wash all vegetables and fruits you use to remove traces of insecticides and fertilisers.

Ready-made juices

Many manufacturers add preservatives or additives to packaged or bottled juices. Often, however, these are naturally occurring plant by-products and not necessarily harmful. By far the most common added ingredient in juice is refined sugar.

If you buy ready-made juices or the frozen concentrates, read the label to make sure that they have no added sugar or colourings, especially if you are giving them to children. For younger children, even pure fruit juices should always be diluted; many juices are quite acidic and can damage young teeth or cause diarrhoea if children drink them at full strength.

JUICES AND THEIR NUTRIENTS

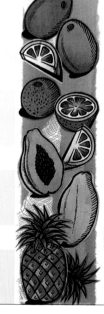

BEETROOT (COOKED)

Beta carotene, folic acid, magnesium, potassium, calcium, iron.

CARROT

Beta carotene, folic acid, potassium, magnesium, phosphorus.

CRANBERRY

Vitamin C, beta carotene, folic acid, magnesium, potassium.

GRAPE

Vitamin C (if fortified), magnesium, phosphorus, potassium.

MANGO

Beta carotene, vitamin C, magnesium, potassium.

ORANGE

Vitamin C, beta carotene, folic acid, magnesium, calcium, phosphorus.

PAPAYA

Vitamin C, beta carotene, phosphorus, potassium.

PINEAPPLE

Vitamin C, folic acid, magnesium.

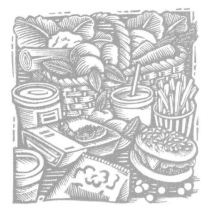

HEALTHY AND HARMFUL FOODS

*In the last few years, there has
been a growing awareness, backed up by
worldwide research, that some kinds of food
may protect against disease or form part of the cure,
while an excess of other types of food can contribute
to problems such as cancer, heart disease, obesity,
and tooth decay. In addition, new farming and
processing techniques, an increased consumption
of convenience foods and fast foods and a series
of 'food scares' – all these have caused growing
concern about the health consequences
of the food we eat.*

THE FRESHNESS FACTOR

Processed foods are convenient, but are they healthy? A steady diet of convenience foods may not provide all your nutritional requirements, but some of these foods do have benefits.

THE FRESHEST WAY

Although the nutritional value of fresh produce diminishes between harvesting and sale, you can still get the best from your food if you:

▶ *Shop for fresh produce frequently rather than once a week.*

▶ *Buy local produce that is in season.*

▶ *Use vegetables and fruits as soon as possible. If you cannot use them immediately, store root vegetables and onions unwashed in a dark, well-ventilated cupboard. Store other vegetables in the refrigerator.*

SCRUBBING VEGETABLES The peel and the layer under it contains valuable nutrients, so scrub vegetables clean rather than peeling them. But do cut out green spots from potato skins.

From peaches to pork to ready-to-eat meals, an extensive range of foods is treated in different ways to prevent decay. Foods are subjected to heat or cold, irradiation and chemical processes to overcome seasonal fluctuations and make them more widely available.

A 1987 British Social Attitudes survey found that 86 per cent of adults interviewed had made an effort to change to a healthier diet over the last ten years. Of these, 57 per cent claimed they had cut down on sugar, 56 per cent grilled rather than fried food, 56 per cent ate more wholemeal bread, 37 per cent had cut down on processed meats, and 27 per cent ate more fresh fruit and vegetables. While these are impressive numbers, it has been estimated that ready-prepared or processed foods still make up between 75 to 80 per cent of most people's diets.

A well-balanced diet should include all the vitamins and minerals the body needs to function properly, plus protein to build and maintain muscle mass; fats and carbohydrates for energy; and fibre to aid bowel function. The concern over processed foods is that they may not provide this balance if they are the only types of foods you eat.

MISSING NUTRIENTS

During processing, foods lose some essential vitamins and minerals. When vegetables, for example, are heated in the canning process, their content of vitamins B and C is reduced.

NUTRITIONAL CONTENT OF FRESH AND PROCESSED FOOD

PRODUCT	QUANTITY	CALORIES	PROTEIN (grams)	CARBOHYDRATE (grams)	FAT (grams)	SODIUM (milligrams)
CHICKEN						
Roast with skin	115 g (4 oz)	248	26	0	16.1	83
Roast without skin	115 g (4 oz)	170	29	0	6.2	93
Canned	115 g (4 oz)	260	14	0	20	1216
PEACH						
Fresh	1	31	0.6	9.7	0.1	3
Canned slices in syrup	55 g (2 oz)	33	0	8.4	0	2
Frozen slices	55 g (2 oz)	118	0.8	30	0.2	8
POTATO						
Boiled	115 g (4 oz)	86	1.7	20	0.3	10
Canned	115 g (4 oz)	72	1.7	17	0.1	287
Dried flakes rehydrated	115 g (4 oz)	81	2.3	18	0.1	299
PEAS						
Fresh	115 g (4 oz)	95	8	11.5	1.7	trace
Canned	115 g (4 oz)	92	6	15.5	1	288
Frozen	115 g (4 oz)	80	6.9	11	1	2.5

Although minerals are not affected by heating, they leach into the canning liquid. Therefore, minerals such as magnesium and zinc can be reduced by up to 50 per cent if the liquid is not consumed. Canned vegetables lose further vitamins if they are stored for more than a year, unless the storage temperature is less than 18.3°C (65°F).

The canning process, however, effectively protects food from food-poisoning microbes like bacteria and fungi. To help retain nutrients leached from foods, use the liquid from canned vegetables in soups and stews.

Unfortunately, some precooked frozen meals also lose nutrients through reheating. Even the best quality precooked foods tend to be low in vitamin C.

The problem with processed foods is not only what is lost but what is added. Some processed produce tends to be high in unhealthy additives such as salt and sugar. Dishes with sauces and pastry are usually high in saturated fats and also low in fibre.

HOW FRESH IS 'FRESH' FOOD?

There is a difference between garden-fresh and market-fresh foods. Foods that are sold as 'fresh' may not be as wholesome as they appear. Much fresh fruit comes from abroad or from across the country and has spent days or weeks in transit and storage. Even locally harvested vegetables are often stored before they are sold. The moment a fruit or vegetable is picked, it starts losing nutrients because it continues to respire and exhaust its nutrient supply. Ideally, fruits and vegetables should be eaten the same day they are harvested. Unfortunately, this is rarely possible unless you grow your own.

Frozen fruits and vegetables, however, can be just as nutritious as fresh. Because they are invariably harvested at peak quality and quick-frozen, they retain nearly all of their food value. In fact, frozen fruit may keep more of its vitamin C than fresh fruit, which continues to respire and is subjected to possible injury in transport and storage.

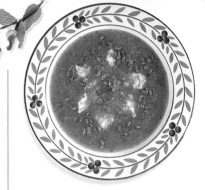

QUICK AND NOURISHING
A tasty pea soup can be made with 115 g (4 oz) of frozen peas, 1 onion, water, half 1 small head of lettuce, 1 tbsp mint, 1 tsp olive oil and topped with 1 tbsp plain yoghurt. This compares favourably with the same quantity of canned pea soups. The fresh soup has only 16 mg of sodium, while the canned soup has 1550 mg.

PROCESSED FISH

An important source of protein and other nutrients in the diet, fish is not widely available fresh. Many species are caught far from where they are consumed, and these are processed for preservation in a variety of ways. Most fish are canned in vegetable oils that are low in saturated fats (see p. 50).

Frozen fish should be solid with no chips of ice in the packaging

Cod fillets

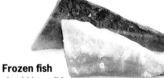

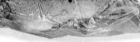

Trout

Choose canned fish that are packed in brine if you are concerned about the fat content of your diet

Sardines in brine

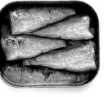

Sardines in oil

Sardines in tomato sauce

Haddock

Fish stays uncooked as it is cold-smoked

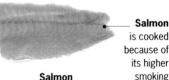

Salmon is cooked because of its higher smoking temperature

Salmon

FROZEN FISH
This is not only quick and easy to cook but retains much of its original nutritional value. Such fish are usually prepared and frozen on the fishing trawlers when they are in peak condition. Products include whole fish, fillets, breaded fish, shellfish and ready-prepared dishes that only need reheating. When choosing frozen fish, check for discoloration – an indication that the fish may have thawed and been refrozen.

CANNED FISH
Some oil-rich fish and shellfish are preserved by canning – packed in oil, brine or tomato sauce. With their high-protein content, canned sardines, salmon, tuna, crab meat and mussels provide nutritious meals or snacks. Oil-rich fish are a valuable source of omega-3 fatty acids that help to reduce the risk of heart disease (see p. 53). Eating canned salmon and sardines with their bones will provide a good intake of calcium.

SMOKED FISH
Certain fish, like haddock and salmon, are preserved by smoking, that is they are salted before being hung in an oven or kiln where smoke from burning hardwood is blown over them for varying periods of time. The chemical properties of smoke are such that smoked fish should be consumed only occasionally. The salt content of smoked fish can vary (see label for amount) and may not be suitable for people on low-salt diets.

Dried fruit

For a ready supply of this delicious snack, dry your own fresh fruit in an oven. Choose firm fruit that is just ripe. Berries can be left whole, but peel, core and thinly slice other fruits. To prevent fruits such as apples from darkening, brush them with lemon juice and water. A convection oven is preferred for drying because its fan will circulate the air. If you are using a conventional oven, prop open the door and set a fan nearby to blow air into the oven. Make sure the room is well ventilated. Keep the oven temperature between 49°C and 60°C (120°F and 140°F). Place the fruit on baking trays and rotate them from time to time. When the fruit is ready, it will feel malleable and leathery. Special dehydrators for fruit are also available.

GETTING IT RIGHT

If a diet high in processed foods is supplemented with several daily servings of fresh fruits and vegetables, the body manages to get all the nutrients it needs. But this does not mean that the diet is healthy or balanced – it may still contain too much fat, salt and sugar, and too little fibre if wholegrain cereals and breads are omitted and too many snacks or desserts are eaten. But since time for shopping, preparing and cooking fresh foods is limited for many people, processed foods may play a helpful role without posing a risk to good health. With careful selection, some processed foods such as wholemeal bread, canned sardines, frozen vegetables and low-fat milk may be nutritionally valuable as well as convenient.

PROCESSING AND PACKAGING

Food preservation methods include adding chemicals, drying, freezing, heating, irradiating, refining and fermenting. Then the food is packed in anything from a steel or an aluminium can to a cardboard box or a cling-film wrapped container. There is some concern, however, that these processes damage the food they are designed to protect.

Irradiation

Of all the preserving techniques, irradiation has aroused the most fear. People are worried that the food may be radioactive and

that it can be life-threatening. But in fact irradiated food is not radioactive, and the doses of radiation used have been approved as safe by the United Nations Joint Committee on Food Irradiation.

Irradiation works by exposing food to a dose of gamma rays from a radioactive source. The rays kill both the disease-causing and other bacteria that occur naturally in many foods, preventing them from accumulating and producing toxins. Low doses of radiation can prevent sprouting in potatoes. The technique also slows the ripening process in fruits and vegetables, and so increases their shelf life.

Not all foods benefit from irradiation. Fats, for example, may be mixed with oxygen (oxidised) and become more susceptible to rancidness. For this reason, irradiation is not used for most milk products and fatty or oily food, such as sardines. In Britain, by law, all foods that have been irradiated must be labelled to indicate this.

Another important concern with irradiation is nutrient loss. Among the vitamins that can be damaged are A, the B group including folic acid, and C, E and K. Depending on the food, however, vitamin losses are about the same as the loss through preparation and cooking. But irradiation may cause an acceleration in the loss of some vitamins during storage because less refrigeration is necessary.

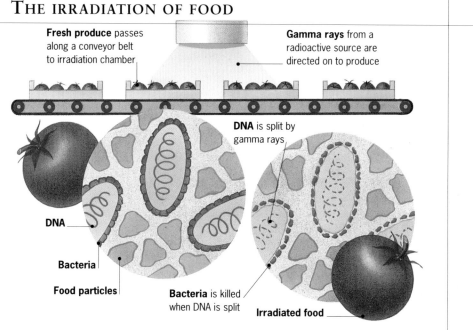

THE IRRADIATION OF FOOD

Tomatoes and many other fresh fruits and vegetables are irradiated to destroy bacteria and delay the ripening process. This reduces the need for preservatives and additives and helps to maintain the look of the food during distribution and storage.

INCREASING THE SHELF LIFE
To irradiate food, gamma rays from a radioactive source are directed onto packaged food. The rays pass through the food, splitting the DNA (genetic material) of the food's natural bacteria, thus killing the bacteria.

Fresh produce passes along a conveyor belt to irradiation chamber

Gamma rays from a radioactive source are directed on to produce

DNA is split by gamma rays

DNA

Bacteria

Food particles

Bacteria is killed when DNA is split

Irradiated food

Freezing

In contrast to irradiation, freezing is one of the best ways to preserve the nutritional content of food. Fewer nutrients are lost by freezing than with any other method of preserving. Freezing stops the activity of bacteria and enzymes, which cause vitamin loss, because the water in the food is bound as ice. However, the bacteria and enzymes are not destroyed and can become active again when the food thaws.

Freezing, however, can affect the flavour and texture of some foods, especially if they are not rapidly frozen or are subjected to refreezing. The flavour of garlic and green pepper strengthens, while that of onions weakens, for example. Sage develops a bitter taste. Fried foods tend to taste stale.

Safe packaging

Some forms of packaging may taint food. In particular, fears have been raised over the safety of cling film. Supermarkets sell many foods, such as meat, cheeses, sandwiches, fruits and vegetables wrapped in this stretchy polyvinyl-chloride (PVC) product. Plasticisers are added to the PVC to make it cling, and the possibility of these plasticisers migrating into the wrapped foods causes concern.

The National Toxicology Program in the United States was the first to publish findings showing that plasticisers could cause cancer in test animals. In Britain, the Ministry of Agriculture, Fisheries and Food (MAFF) initiated research that revealed the plasticiser known as di-2-ethylhexyl, or DEHA – which is thought to cause cancer – was eight times more likely to end up in food than other plasticisers. Migration was at its worst with tightly wrapped, high-fat products like salami, pork and beef. The biggest absorption of plasticisers occurred in foods that had been wrapped in cling film and then cooked in a microwave oven.

Although the threat to health posed by cling film is not yet clear, avoid placing products containing DEHA in microwaves. If possible, choose products that are labelled 'Non-PVC' or 'Plasticiser-free' or remove the food from shop containers and rewrap in plastic bags at home.

Aluminium

Another suspect packaging material is aluminium. Research conducted in the United Kingdom and United States has shown that aluminium may be a danger to the elderly, particularly people with kidney disorders. It also may be a contributory factor in anaemia and Alzheimer's disease. It is possible, but highly unlikely, that aluminium can enter the body through foods that are packed in aluminium cans or cooked in aluminium foil or saucepans (see p. 74).

ORGANIC PRODUCE

Fears about adulterated produce and the effects of intensive farming on the environment have led to the increasing popularity of organic, or 'green', foods.

USING CLING FILM SAFELY

Covering dishes of food to be cooked in a microwave oven will help to retain moisture. Steam will be produced that helps to speed the food's cooking time. Always use microwave-safe, non-PVC cling film.

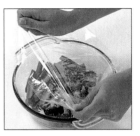

ALLOWING SPACE
When covering a dish with cling film, do not let it touch the food.

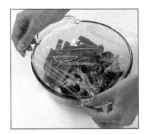

VENTING CLING FILM
Steam can split the cling film, so turn back a corner to form an opening, which will allow steam to escape.

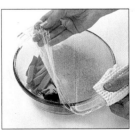

AVOIDING BURNS
To avoid getting burned when removing the cling film, lift the edge farthest from you and then carefully peel it towards you.

DRYING METHODS

Originally, foods such as dates and grapes and strips of meat or fish were spread out in the sun to dry. Meat and fish were also smoked to dry them. Modern drying methods, however, are varied and allow more types of food to be dried. Some fruits and vegetables are tunnel-dried; they are placed in a tunnel and exposed to blasts of hot air until their moisture content is reduced to 25 per cent. Potatoes, milk and eggs may be dehydrated until they retain only two to ten per cent moisture.

Accelerated freeze-drying involves a process that removes moisture from food after it has been frozen. This process is used to make instant coffee and the freeze-dried fruits and vegetables used by campers. The flavour and colour of these products, when reconstituted, are often of good quality, comparing well to the fresh food.

DRIED FOODS
The oldest method of preserving food, drying removes water from food and thereby stops bacterial growth and inhibits enzyme activity.

KEEPING ORGANIC FOOD SAFE

The likelihood of lower chemical residues may make organic food safer to eat, but there are still some precautions needed when selecting, using and storing such foods.

▶ *Look for a symbol that guarantees the product has met stringent organic guidelines – for example, the Soil Association symbol in the UK.*

▶ *Just before you use them, wash all fruits and vegetables under cold running water.*

▶ *To avoid rancidness, store food rich in nuts, seeds and oils in the refrigerator rather than a cupboard. Do not keep them for more than a few weeks.*

▶ *Follow strict guidelines when canning or bottling produce, whether conventional or organic.*

Organic farmers grow crops without using chemical fertilisers or pesticides. To do this, they use traditional techniques such as mixed farming (planting two or more crops in the same field), crop rotation (planting different crops in sequence), shallow ploughing, and fertilising with animal manure, together with complex products like seaweed fertilisers and methods such as natural biological pest control. In any subsequent processing, no further additives or preservatives are used.

Is organic food better?

Its supporters claim that organic produce is more nutritious, has a better taste and texture, and because it contains no residues from pesticides and fertilisers, is better for you. It is important to recognise that the organic methods used function because of naturally occurring toxins on which there is little or no scientific data. But whether organic produce is healthier than conventional produce depends on whether the amounts and levels of chemical products used in intensive farming really do cause any long-term effects on human health. Tests are still being conducted on many agricultural chemicals and, consequently, it is difficult to make definitive statements about their levels of safety.

The regulation of pesticides

History, however, suggests there may be some justification for concern about modern agricultural practices. The pesticide

DDT was developed in the late 1930s and introduced in 1945. By 1972 it was outlawed in the United States after it was found to have damaging effects on the human nervous system. It was withdrawn from sale in Britain in 1984. Subsequently, all chemical products used in food production have come under scrutiny. However, DDT is still used in many developing countries.

In the United Kingdom, the Ministry of Agriculture, Fisheries and Food (MAFF) has approved the use of 450 pesticide ingredients. The UK Pesticides Directorate (PSD) assert that "pesticide manufacturers are required to provide a wide range of scientific data, which are subject to rigorous scrutiny by the independent experts on the Advisory Committee on Pesticides". Only when products are shown to pose no unacceptable risk will approval be given for them to be put on the market. Newer pesticides are not persistent and, if used properly, do not lead to detectable residues in foods.

Maximum residue limits (MRL) have been set for some fruit and vegetables to assure minimal risk, and reviews are under way on the 250 pesticides licensed for use in the United Kingdom before 1981. By July 1994, 106 evaluations had been published by the PSD. The European Commission is also conducting a review programme of about 800 substances. This programme should be completed by 2003.

Pesticide limits are strict in the United States. But in 1988 the National Academy of Science noted that "some allowed levels

---

A DIFFERENT LOOK

Organic foods may please the palate, but they do not always tempt the eye because of blemishes and irregular shapes. They may also have insect residues (which should be washed off) and a strong aroma.

CONVENTIONAL PRODUCE
Many genetically altered foods are said to have a designer look that may appeal to consumers, but that does not assure the food's nutritional value.

Apples are often waxed for a shiny appearance

Pesticides on conventional produce often leave residues on the outer surface of foods

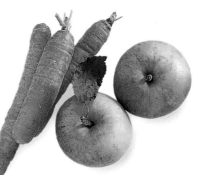

ORGANIC PRODUCE
The seeming imperfections of organic produce are harmless and do not affect the food's taste or nutritional value.

[of pesticide residues in food] are being challenged by scientists as being too high". The Food and Drug Administration (FDA), however, routinely monitors the chemicals in foods. Any farmer who exceeds the pesticide limits in fruits and vegetables faces legal action, fines and possibly the loss of crops. But the FDA rarely discovers cases in which the pesticide limits are violated.

It is possible that the delayed effects on human health from synthetic pesticides and fertilisers are sufficiently small to be of no consequence. But until the investigations into all the modern farmers' chemical aids are complete, doubts may remain.

ARE THERE PERFECT FOODS?

To ensure a well-balanced diet, you normally need to eat a combination of foods. There are some foods, however, which contain such a wide range of essential nutrients that they may be considered almost perfect. Three such foods – wheat, bananas and milk – are packed with so much goodness they seem to be in a class of their own.

WHEAT

Sometimes called the 'staff of life', wheat provides anywhere from 15 to 60 per cent of the calories and protein in most people's diets. Of the 44 known essential nutrients, only five are missing from wheat – vitamins A, B_{12}, C and D, and iodine. The wheat

> ### CAUTION
> *Organic produce lacks the preservatives present in ordinary foods, so always check to make sure the food is completely fresh. Mouldy food (a major source of potent carcinogens) can pose a serious health risk.*

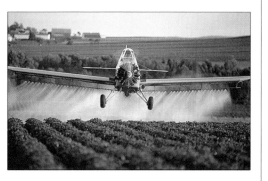

INTENSIVE FARMING
Fewer farmers now rely heavily on chemical fertilisers and pesticides. More farmers are using integrated pest management with much lower applications of chemicals. Using chemical products, however, ensures a high crop yield and wards off spoilage, making food more widely available and cheaper for the consumer.

berry contains 22 vitamins and minerals, protein and dietary fibre but the protein is not a complete protein. To get complete

AVOIDING RISKS OF PESTICIDES

If organic produce is not easily available, try adopting some of these measures to minimise the possible dangers of pesticides and other chemicals that can be found in conventionally grown foods.

▶ *Eat a wide variety of foods. This reduces exposure to any one pesticide.*

▶ *Eat seasonal produce. Imported or domestically grown out-of-season vegetables and fruit are more likely to have been encouraged to grow chemically.*

▶ *Choose local or domestically grown produce. Imported food – particularly from developing countries – is often grown under less stringent controls on chemical use.*

▶ *Wash vegetables and fruit just before eating. Surface residues are often water-soluble and can be rinsed away.*

▶ *Peel any produce that has a shiny coating or buy unwaxed organic produce. Surface residues are sealed in by the wax.*

▶ *Trim vegetables and fruit. Residues tend to be concentrated in the tops and outer leaves of vegetables.*

▶ *Grow your own produce. There is a range of safe non-chemical pest control methods for the home gardener.*

ORGANIC WINE

A glass of wine can be even more enjoyable if it is low in artificial additives. It may be less likely to give you a reaction if you are sensitive to sulfites (see p. 105).

Organic wine is made from grapes grown without chemical fertilisers and pesticides. During winemaking only low levels of sulphur dioxide are allowed, reducing the chances of an allergic reaction in people who suffer from asthma or bronchial problems.

To identify organic wines, look for an organic organisation's symbol on the label. French bottles may also be labelled with a description such as "*Ce vin est cultive sans engrais chimiques, sans insecticide*" or "*Production de l'agriculture biologique*".

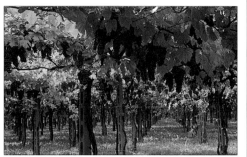

ORGANIC VINEYARD
Vines that are free from chemical fertilisers and pesticides can yield wines as high in quality as those from the most cultured grape. The quality of organic wines is as varied as that of ordinary wines. Their flavour and character are usually similar to those of conventionally produced wines of the same grape variety and region.

A grain of wheat

The wheat berry is a rich source of nutrients. The bran, five or six layers of protective coating, mainly consists of fibre. It also has a high proportion of B vitamins, some minerals, and protein. The germ of the wheat, which is the plant embryo, contains polyunsaturated fat, many B vitamins, vitamin E, and protein. The endosperm supplies food to the growing seed. It is mainly composed of starch granules and protein, and has some B vitamins.

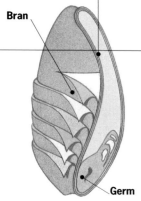

UNREFINED WHEAT
The most nutritious wholemeal flour is stone ground as it retains most of the original wheat berry.

protein, wheat needs to be combined with a complementary protein food, such as dried beans, lentils or nuts.

Is wholemeal flour better than plain?

The nutrients in wheat are not evenly distributed throughout the wheat berry. Many of them are concentrated in the outer layers (bran) and in the germ (the tiny seed at the bottom of the kernel), both of which are lost when wheat is refined.

Refined wheat flour has 60 to 80 per cent fewer nutrients than the whole kernel and only ten per cent of its fibre. Given these figures, the nutritional benefits of eating wholewheat products are obvious.

Is wheat fattening?

Wheat has suffered some bad publicity in the past. It was thought that its carbohydrate content made it fattening. The truth is that carbohydrates are an important energy source, and they are particularly valuable when they come in the natural form of whole grains. It is not the wheat itself but the butter, creamy sauces and oily spreads that people put on bread and other wheat products, such as pasta, that are fattening.

BANANAS

At 123 calories and almost no fat, a banana is an ideal between-meal snack and energy booster, as the many tennis players who eat them between sets can affirm. Bananas contain a large amount of potassium, a mineral that helps to control blood pressure and heart function, thus protecting against heart attack, stroke and irregular heart rhythms. Bananas also contain 30 per cent of the recommended daily requirement of vitamin B_6, and 20 per cent of vitamin C.

MILK

Milk is an important source of nourishment at most stages of life. Essential for developing children's bones and teeth, milk can also

> ### C A U T I O N
> *Children should not be given semi-skimmed milk before two years of age and then only if they are eating a varied diet. Skimmed milk should not be given to children under five years of age.*

maintain health in adulthood and even into old age. Milk is a rich source of calcium and supplies other important minerals, notably zinc, magnesium, potassium and phosphorus. It also contains high-quality protein, and a wide range of vitamins – A, B_1, B_2, B_6, B_{12}, and, when fortified, D. Carbohydrate is present in the form of a simple disaccharide, lactose (milk sugar). Whole milk is also high in saturated fat, but by choosing semi-skimmed or skimmed milk you can enjoy the benefits of milk without going overboard on fat.

Although milk contains an abundance of many important nutrients, it is not a 'complete' food. Milk lacks fibre and is a poor source of dietary iron and vitamin C. After the first few months of an infant's life, even breast milk needs to be augmented with other foods to produce a balanced diet.

The importance of calcium

Healthy growth and the maintenance of bones and teeth depend on a good supply of calcium (as well as zinc, copper, manganese, fluoride and protein). Blood pressure is also influenced by calcium. American research has shown that children with the highest intake of calcium have the lowest blood pressure. Calcium is particularly important for girls and women. Adolescent girls who get little calcium may compromise the growth of their bone mass. In later life they are more apt to suffer from osteoporosis, a gradual thinning of the bone structure that may result in fractures. Pregnant and breast-

NUTRIENT CONTENT OF FLOUR (PER 115 G/4 OZ)

FLOUR	CALORIES	PROTEIN (grams)	CARBOHYDRATE (grams)	FAT (grams)	SODIUM (milligrams)	FIBRE (grams)
Wholemeal	357	14.6	73	2.5	4	10.4
White, plain	392	10.8	89	1.5	4	4
Self-raising	380	10.2	87	1.4	414	3.6

WHAT MILK IS BEST?

Because of the differences in processing, milk differs in composition and nutritional value. Look at the label for help in choosing the right one for your diet. Most of the milk sold is pasteurised. Because the milk is heated to 72°C (162°F) to kill bacteria, B vitamins are reduced by 10 per cent and vitamin C by 25 per cent.

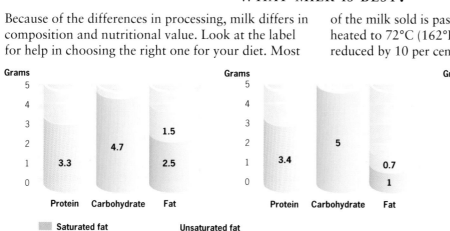

WHOLE MILK
The average fat content of pasteurised whole milk is 3.5 per cent.
A 100 millilitre (3.5 fluid ounce) serving of whole milk consists of 3.3 grams of protein, 4.7 grams of carbohydrate and 4 grams of fat, of which 2.5 grams are saturated.

SEMI-SKIMMED
When milk is semi-skimmed, it retains only a 2 per cent fat content – it also loses a proportion of vitamin A and D content. 100 millilitres (3.5 fluid ounces) of semi-skimmed milk consists of 3.4 grams of protein, 5 grams of carbohydrate and 1.7 grams of fat, of which 1 gram is saturated. Semi-skimmed milk is not suitable for children under two years.

SKIMMED
Milk that is skimmed has almost no fat – less than 0.5 per cent. It retains the calcium of whole milk, but loses more vitamin A and D with the fat. 100 millilitres (3.5 fluid ounces) of skimmed milk contains 3.4 grams of protein, 5 grams of carbohydrate and 0.1 gram of fat, of which 0.06 of a gram is saturated. Skimmed milk is not suitable for children under five years.

feeding women require calcium to support foetal and infant growth. During the menopause, increased calcium intake may help to counteract loss of bone mass because of a drop in oestrogen levels.

Children under the age of 11 should drink at least two to three glasses of milk a day; teenagers and young adults, four cups; older adults, two to three cups; breastfeeding mothers and postmenopausal women, four cups or more. Choose low-fat milks for everybody over the age of five (see p. 50).

Milk allergies
Not everyone can drink milk. Some people – especially Asians, Eskimos, Africans, Native Americans and up to 40 per cent of Caucasians – lack sufficient amounts of the enzyme lactase in their intestines to break down the lactose in milk (see p. 108). For those people, milk with a reduced lactose content is available. Alternatively, lactose-intolerant people can try eating yoghurt, which has less lactose than milk but still contains plenty of protein and milk nutrients and is a more concentrated source of calcium (see p. 102).

THE IDEAL FOOD
Breast milk is undoubtedly best for babies. It is free, does not need sterilising, is the proper temperature, and contains just the right amount of proteins, vitamins and minerals a growing baby needs.

In addition, breast milk contains important antibodies that provide the baby with a natural protection against viral illnesses, respiratory infection and infections of the gastrointestinal tract.

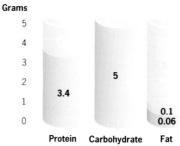

Breast milk supplies the baby with 70 calories per 100 ml (3.5 fl oz)

SATISFYING A BABY'S NEEDS
Breast milk provides a baby with essential nutrients. Some nutrients, such as iron and vitamin D, are absorbed much more efficiently from breast milk than from formula milk.

HEALTHFUL FOODS

Research has shown that certain foods contain special nutrients, chemical compounds and even bacteria that can help to prevent certain diseases, relieve health complaints and boost energy.

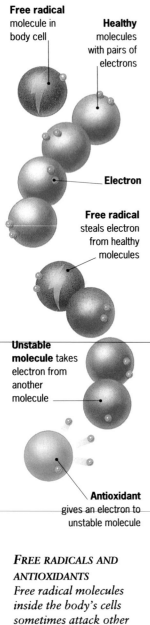

Free radical
molecule in
body cell

Healthy
molecules
with pairs of
electrons

Electron

Free radical
steals electron
from healthy
molecules

**Unstable
molecule** takes
electron from
another
molecule

Antioxidant
gives an electron to
unstable molecule

*FREE RADICALS AND
ANTIOXIDANTS
Free radical molecules
inside the body's cells
sometimes attack other
molecules by taking an
electron. The healthy
molecule, in turn,
becomes a free radical
and attacks another
molecule, removing its
electron. A chain
reaction is started,
which is broken when
an antioxidant is present.
The antioxidant, not
requiring two electrons,
gives one to the
unstable molecule.*

The evidence from more than 300 studies has revealed that fruits and vegetables offer powerful protection against disease. It appears that the vegetables with the most effective weapon against cancer and other diseases are the crucifers, or cabbage family, which include broccoli. These vegetables contain anticancer substances known as antioxidants, which attack molecules called free radicals.

Free radicals are released in all cells as part of the body's normal biochemistry and defence mechanism against disease. Free radicals occur as a response to everyday living – exposure to ultraviolet light waves and environmental pollutants such as motor vehicle emissions. If free radicals become too numerous, however, they attack the body itself. It is believed that unchecked free radical action can lead to premature ageing and, through damage to DNA (genetic material), some forms of cancer.

THE BENEFITS OF ANTIOXIDANTS

Stable molecules in the body have pairs of electrons, but free radicals have at least one that is unpaired; this makes them unstable.

To achieve stability, free radicals steal electrons from other molecules, thereby making them unstable. The remaining molecule, which is now a free radical, sets off to take another electron from a complete molecule. A destructive chain reaction is thus set in motion. Antioxidants are substances that negate the harmful effects of free radicals by providing them with an electron, but do not become unstable themselves. The antioxidants then are safely broken down and absorbed by the body.

The main antioxidants are the carotenes, especially beta carotene (the plant source of vitamin A found in carrots and oranges); vitamins C and E; the minerals selenium, zinc and magnesium; and protein, in particular glutathione, which is a combination of three amino acids – glutamate, glycine, and cysteine. These are found in the cruciferous family and many other fruits and vegetables, such as bananas and peas.

The antioxidants that have been subject to the most study are beta carotene, vitamin C and vitamin E. In American trials, a high dietary intake of beta carotene has been associated with a reduced risk of both heart

---

HEALTHY HERB

Parsley is a member of the umbellifer family, which, like the crucifer family, is being investigated for its disease-fighting properties. This biennial plant contains beta carotene and vitamin C, which may protect against cancers and heart disease, and boost the immune system.

*USING PARSLEY
There are several types of parsley, but the two best-known are curly-leaved parsley and flat-leaved (Italian) parsley. Parsley leaves offer B vitamins, iron, calcium, magnesium*

and fibre, as well as antioxidants. They can be added to a variety of dishes, including stews, salads, baked potatoes and peas, or used as an edible garnish. Chewing raw parsley leaves can help to freshen breath.

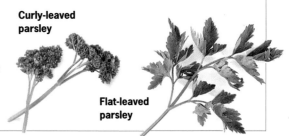

**Curly-leaved
parsley**

**Flat-leaved
parsley**

disease and cancers of the mouth, throat, oesophagus, larynx, lungs, stomach, cervix and bladder. Other studies have discovered a relationship between a high dietary intake of vitamin C, found in oranges, sweet peppers and many other fruits and vegetables, and a reduced risk of cataracts and heart disease. A high consumption of vitamin E, found in vegetable oils, sunflower seeds and a variety of nuts, has been linked to a reduced risk of gastrointestinal cancer, lung cancer and thrombosis.

No match for nicotine

Antioxidants may help to protect the body from many illnesses, but they are no match for the effects of tobacco. A study of 29 000 long-term Finnish smokers, all over the age of 50, by The National Cancer Institute in the United States and Finland's National Public Health Institute found that regular doses of vitamin E and beta carotene did not lessen smokers' chances of suffering lung cancer or stroke. In fact, those who took the antioxidants had a higher incidence of these illnesses than a similar group of men who took nothing. The researchers were puzzled by these unexpected results and are still analysing them. It is possible that cancer was already in progress and that antioxidants are preventative rather than therapeutic agents.

> **CAUTION**
> *Some of the disease-fighting abilities of phytochemicals and antioxidants are destroyed by overcooking. To get the most good from vegetables, eat them raw, lightly cooked or microwaved.*

PHYTOCHEMICALS

Discovered in 1978, phytochemicals are being hailed as the new hope in the ongoing fight against cancer. Phytochemicals – and there are literally thousands of them present in vegetables and fruits – are neither vitamins nor minerals but rather chemical compounds that evolved to protect plants from injury and disease. In humans, phytochemicals seem to act as potent cancer inhibitors or stimulators of natural mechanisms to inactivate noxious compounds. One group of vegetables, the cruciferous family, is particularly rich in these chemicals, but other vegetables and fruits, such as corn and citrus fruits, also contain many important phytochemicals.

How do phytochemicals work?

Researchers in the United States found that if the phytochemical sulforaphane is added to human cells growing in a laboratory dish,

Anticancer foods

Antioxidants and phytochemicals are found in all fruits and vegetables. In addition to crucifers (the cabbage family), the following foods contain anticancer agents: asparagus, bananas, carrots, celery, corn-on-the-cob, dates, figs, garlic, grapes, grapefruit, kiwifruit, onions, oranges, peas, pumpkins, soya beans, sweet potatoes and tomatoes.

PHYTOCHEMICALS

Sulforaphane, a phytochemical found in cruciferous vegetables, helps to prevent cells from developing cancer. It seems that within only hours of being eaten, sulforaphane enters the bloodstream and triggers a self-defence system in the body. This acts to detoxify carcinogens. Research is currently being carried out on developing a synthetic version of sulforaphane, but brussels sprouts are a prime natural source.

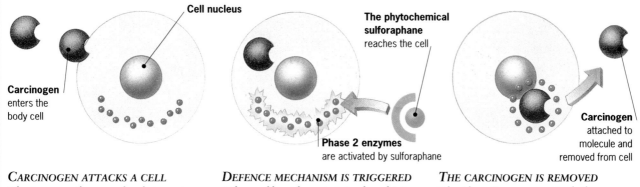

CARCINOGEN ATTACKS A CELL
The process of cancer development starts when a carcinogenic molecule or mutagen enters a cell.

DEFENCE MECHANISM IS TRIGGERED
When sulforaphane is introduced into the body, it activates phase 2 enzymes, which are naturally occurring cancer fighting proteins in the cell.

THE CARCINOGEN IS REMOVED
The phase 2 enzymes attach the carcinogen to a molecule, which carries it away from the cell.

CANCER-PREVENTING VEGETABLES

The cabbages and other green, leafy vegetables are a valuable accompaniment to a meal. Use them raw in salads, cooked on their own and sprinkled with sesame seeds, or cooked with other foods. Eat at least one of these vegetables each day as part of a programme of eating five daily servings of fruits and vegetables. But do not restrict your intake to just one member of the cabbage family, as they all contain important nutrients.

VEGETABLE	CHOOSING	STORING	USING
BROCCOLI The star of the crucifer family, broccoli is abundant in beta carotene, vitamin C, potassium, calcium, folic acid and several phytochemicals.	The florets should be crisp and tightly closed. They should be a dark green or purplish colour. Avoid any with brown or spotted stems.	Refrigerate, unwashed, in an open plastic bag. The broccoli will keep for about four days. Once cooked, store in a tightly covered container for up to three days.	Wash thoroughly under cold running water. Cut the stalks a few inches below the florets, and pierce the bottom of each stalk for even cooking.
BRUSSELS SPROUTS Brussels sprouts are rich sources of sulforaphane and other phytochemicals and antioxidants. They are one of the best vegetable sources of dietary fibre.	The vegetables should be bright green and firm, with tight heads. Choose sprouts of a similar size for even cooking. Avoid any with yellow leaves.	Refrigerate, unwashed, in a perforated plastic bag for up to five days.	Rinse thoroughly. Trim stem ends. Cut an 'X' in the bottom of each stem for even cooking.
CABBAGE The many varieties of cabbage contain numerous antioxidant compounds. Chinese cabbage (pak choi) is a particularly rich source of beta carotene, vitamin C, potassium and calcium.	Cabbage heads should have only three or four loose outer leaves that are pliable but not limp. Avoid heads with damaged leaves or split stems.	Refrigerate in a perforated plastic bag. An uncut cabbage will keep for about two weeks. Once cut, use within a couple of days.	Remove tough outer leaves. Cut the cabbage into quarters, then into wedges, before removing the core. For slicing, retain the core in the wedge to keep leaves from separating.
CAULIFLOWER Cauliflower is rich in vitamin C, potassium, fibre and several phytochemicals.	Cauliflower should have a firm white or creamy head. The outer leaves should be fresh green and crisp. Avoid heads with spots or loose florets.	Refrigerate, unwashed and stem-side up, for up to five days. Ready-cut florets should be used within 24 hours of purchase.	Remove the leaves and cut out the core. Cook the head whole or separate into florets.
SPINACH Spinach contains four times more beta carotene than broccoli and is a source of vitamins C and E. It is rich in fibre. But it contains oxalic acid, a chemical that limits the absorption of iron and calcium.	Leaves should be dark green, fresh and crisp. Avoid spinach that is bruised or crushed. Stems should be thin.	Refrigerate, unwashed, in a plastic bag for up to four days.	Trim stems and wash thoroughly. Spinach that is to be cooked does not need to be dried; the water clinging to the leaves will steam the spinach without additional cooking liquid.

it boosts the synthesis of cancer-fighting enzymes (protein substances that act as catalysts in the body, breaking down food and aiding metabolism). Like a policeman who removes a troublemaker from a peaceful gathering, these enzymes remove potential or actual mutagens and carcinogens from human cells by handcuffing them to a molecule and whisking them away before they can cause any lasting damage.

Phytochemicals use an impressive array of cancer-blocking tactics. Scientists at Cornell University in New York have reported that p-coumaric acid and chlorogenic acid, two phytochemicals that are found in tomatoes as well as other fruits and vegetables, can prevent carcinogens from forming in the first place. Another anticancer tactic of phytochemicals is to close off the capillaries, hair-thin blood vessels that deliver nutrients to developing tumours. But preventing existing cancers from spreading throughout the body (metastasis) is beyond the capability of these phytochemical compounds.

Fighting breast cancer

An overabundance of the hormone oestrogen may stimulate the growth of breast cancer. But recent American research has shown that phytochemicals in food may help to beat this cancer by obstructing the body's absorption of oestrogen. Widely prevalent in the United States and other countries in the West, breast cancer may also be related to high intakes of fat.

A study by New York's Strang-Cornell Cancer Research Laboratory revealed that oestrogen levels fell dramatically in women who consumed a diet high in spinach and cruciferous vegetables, such as red and white cabbage. It is thought that one of the phytochemicals found in cruciferous vegetables – indole-3-carbinol – deactivates potent oestrogens, thus preventing oestrogen-sensitive cells, particularly those in the breast, from developing tumours.

Another potent phytochemical that has been linked to the prevention of breast cancer is sulforaphane (see box, p. 95). Found in cruciferous vegetables as well as carrots, turnips and spring onions, it too speeds up the removal of oestrogen from the body.

Hope for the future?

Research into phytochemicals is still in its infancy, and there has not yet been time for long-term studies on humans to see whether an existing cancer can be retarded or eradicated by a high intake of these compounds. According to many scientists, phytochemical theory dovetails neatly with the results of numerous studies that have linked diets rich in fresh fruits and vegetables with a lower incidence of cancer.

East and West
Women of all ages should include a range of vegetables in their diets, eating plenty of cauliflower, spinach, cabbage and brussels sprouts. Although postmenopausal women may no longer produce oestrogen from their ovaries, there is still some present in body fat.

The traditional Japanese diet consists of large quantities of leafy green vegetables, and the incidence of breast cancer there has always been lower than in the West. More recently, however, the number of cases in Japan has risen dramatically – 58 per cent between 1975 and 1985. Some researchers believe that this rise is due to many Japanese people adopting a Western-style, high-fat diet.

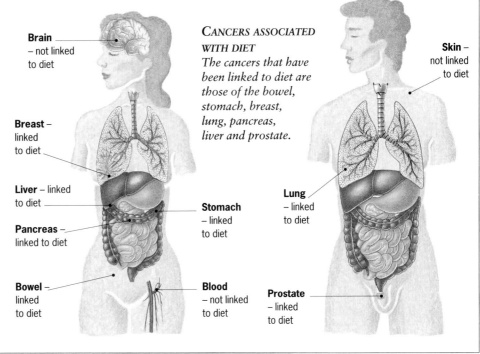

CANCER AND DIET

Some scientists claim that a nutritionally deficient diet is a cause of many cancers. Three factors are thought to play a major role in increasing the possibility of developing cancer: low levels of antioxidants and fibre and high levels of certain kinds of fat.

CANCERS NOT ASSOCIATED WITH DIET
Scientists believe that the following cancers are caused by factors other than diet: brain (often from metastasis from breast or ovarian cancer), skin (too much sun and sunburn), and blood (many factors, including radiation).

CANCERS ASSOCIATED WITH DIET
The cancers that have been linked to diet are those of the bowel, stomach, breast, lung, pancreas, liver and prostate.

Brain – not linked to diet

Breast – linked to diet

Liver – linked to diet

Pancreas – linked to diet

Bowel – linked to diet

Stomach – linked to diet

Blood – not linked to diet

Skin – not linked to diet

Lung – linked to diet

Prostate – linked to diet

Snacks for health
The best type of fruit or vegetable juice is undiluted, with no added sugar. All these drinks provide vitamins that act as antioxidants and some berry drinks prevent bladder infections.

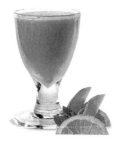

TROPICAL DELIGHT
Freshly squeezed orange juice, blended with mango, provides the antioxidant vitamins C and beta carotene.

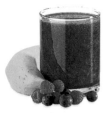

BERRY SURPRISE
Mix cranberries with a sliced banana and some water and blend until smooth. Cranberry juice helps to prevent cystitis.

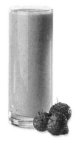

STRAWBERRY SHAKE
Strawberries combined with low-fat milk and plain yoghurt provide a rich blend of vitamin C and calcium.

WHAT ARE THE WONDER FOODS?
Cystitis, herpes, infertility – these three conditions affect thousands of men and women. Could cures lie in simple foods that can be picked in a garden or gathered from the seashore? Over the last few years, there have been many studies to find out whether certain foods have healing properties. In particular, great claims have been made for cranberries, kelp and strawberries.

CRANBERRIES AND CYSTITIS
Regularly drinking a glass of cranberry juice can help to prevent cystitis, a painful urinary infection that has a tendency to recur. The cause of cystitis is the Escherichia coli (*E. coli*) bacteria. Usually existing in the intestines, it can creep into the urinary tract where it sticks to the bladder cells and spreads infection. Symptoms include pain on urination and a frequent need to pass water, as well as abdominal pain and fever. More women than men suffer from cystitis because the opening to the female urethra is closer to the rectum, making it easier for bacteria to enter from the rectal area.

CYSTITIS

One of the main causes of cystitis is *E. coli* bacteria, which normally live harmlessly in the rectum, intestines and on anal skin. It also may be caused by friction on the urethra.

A kidney infection is caused by bacteria travelling up through the ureters

Ureter

A bladder infection occurs when bacteria travelling up from the urethra irritate and inflame the lining of the bladder

A urethral infection is due to bacteria transferred from the intestine multiplying quickly in the urethra

Cranberries have long been used by women as a folk remedy for cystitis. It was thought that the vitamin C in cranberries made the urine more acidic, thereby destroying the bacteria. Then, in 1991, Israeli scientists at the Weizmann Institute of Science discovered two compounds in cranberry juice that cripple the mechanism by which the *E. coli* bacteria attach themselves to the walls of the urinary tract. Denied a firm hold, the bacteria are washed out in the urine, giving the infection no chance to take hold.

What can cranberry juice do?
It appears that from 125 to 450 millilitres (4 to 16 fluid ounces) of cranberry juice can protect against the *E. coli* infection if you are prone to cystitis. A study involving 72 postmenopausal women found that they were 58 per cent less likely to develop bladder infections if they drank 300 millilitres (10 fluid ounces) of cranberry juice a day.

In another study, Prodromos N. Papas of Tufts University School of Medicine in Boston found that drinking 450 millilitres (16 fluid ounces) of cranberry juice a day for three weeks protected 73 per cent of the group from recurring infections. When the women stopped drinking it, half of them suffered a recurrence of the infection within six weeks. But drinking as little as 125 to 175 millilitres (four to six fluid ounces) of cranberry juice a day may be enough to protect against cystitis. This amount prevented bladder infections in two-thirds of a group of 28 men and women taking part in a study in 1991. Bear in mind, however, that cranberry juice has a high sugar content.

Although cranberry juice effectively prevents bladder infections or their recurrence, it should not be used for treating existing infections. If the symptoms are masked, the infection may spread into the kidneys and cause serious problems. If you develop cystitis, stop taking cranberry juice and seek medical advice for its treatment.

KELP AND HERPES
Those people unlucky enough to contract genital herpes are told that the condition is incurable and they will suffer recurring attacks throughout life. The severity of these attacks, however, could be minimised, and possibly even prevented entirely, if recent discoveries in test tube studies of kelp prove just as effective in human trials.

What can kelp do?

Researchers at the University of California put extracts of edible seaweed from the red algae family – generically known as kelp – into test tubes that contained human cells infected with the herpes virus. The spread of the virus slowed by 50 per cent. Also, human cells that were exposed to the kelp extract before being put in with the herpes virus were immune to the infection.

It is not yet known what chemical component in kelp helps to destroy the herpes virus. Kelp contains 13 vitamins, 20 amino acids, 24 trace elements and many phytochemicals. Traditionally, it has been used to treat a variety of complaints, particularly respiratory ailments, digestive disorders and peptic ulcers. But there are health warnings about taking excessive amounts of kelp as it can damage the thyroid gland.

Kelp is available as a supplement in tablet and powder form. The powder can be mixed with water for drinking, or used as a salt substitute. It has a very strong flavour because of its iodine content.

STRAWBERRIES AND SPERM PRODUCTION

According to the latest research on vitamin C intake and healthy sperm, men who are trying to have children may reap benefits from eating strawberries and other fruits and vegetables that contain vitamin C. Just 200 milligrams a day – the amount found in 350 grams (12 ounces) of fresh strawberries – can improve sperm production and viability.

What causes unhealthy sperm?

Falling sperm counts among Western men have been worrying scientists in recent years. Modern-day pollutants and poor diet are among the main causes of low counts. Persistent exposure to toxic compounds, such as those found in air that has been polluted by petrochemicals, can result in those toxins accumulating in the testicles, where the sperm are produced. This can lead to sperm agglutination – a condition in which the sperm clump together after ejaculation and cannot not move around freely – and contributes to infertility. Older men are particularly prone to this condition. A study in which the sperm of 45-year-old men was compared to that of 18-year-olds found that the older men had fewer, less mobile sperm, with a higher incidence of malformation.

ORIENTAL MUSHROOMS

Gourmet cooks love shiitake mushrooms because they add a delightful flavour to many dishes. But health-conscious consumers revere them for their health-giving properties.

Recent studies on laboratory animals show that lentinan, a compound found in these mushrooms, may help to activate the immune system, preventing normal cells from developing into tumours and also counteracting viral infections. But these findings have yet to be supported by studies using humans.

Be very careful when you pick any type of mushrooms. Mushroom poisoning is one of the major causes of plant-derived toxicities. The correct identification of wild mushrooms is critical.

COOKING MUSHROOMS
Shiitake mushrooms are most commonly available dried. Soak them for about 30 minutes in a bowl of water before using in soups or sauces.

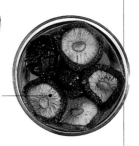

Reconstitute dried shiitake mushrooms

What can vitamin C do?

A 60-day trial on infertile men carried out by Dr William A. Harris at the University of Texas showed that a daily dose of 1 000 milligrams of vitamin C restored fertility to all of the men in the study. Their sperm counts rose by 60 per cent; sperm were 30 per cent livelier, and there were few abnormal sperm. Further tests by Dr Harris and his colleagues showed that just 200 milligrams of vitamin C could produce the same results, although less quickly.

Scientists believe vitamin C is effective against sperm agglutination because of its powerful antioxidant effect. One theory suggests that free radical molecules in the body can attack the protective coating on the sperm's surface causing it to oxidise. The oxidised coating allows the sperm to clump together, which impedes their movement. Vitamin C increases the body's supply of antioxidants, which help to disable the free radicals (see p. 94).

There is no conclusive proof, however, that vitamin C cures male infertility. Factors other than diet may pertain and men with this condition should not rely solely on an increased intake of vitamin C, whether from foods or supplements, to enhance fertility, but should seek medical advice.

STUPENDOUS STRAWBERRIES
As well as being a potent supplier of vitamin C, strawberries contain a natural substance called ellagic acid (also found in other berries, nuts and a number of vegetables) that is said to counteract carcinogens and may help to prevent tumours developing.

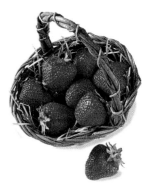

THE ENERGY BOOSTERS

Sugar to boost the body, caffeine to boost the mind – an all-too-familiar response to physical and mental tiredness. But do sugar and caffeine really help or are they actually counterproductive?

Glucose, a simple sugar derived from the carbohydrates in foods, is the body's preferred source of energy. Carbohydrate that is not immediately needed to fuel activity or metabolism is converted into glycogen, then stored in the liver and muscles. If insufficiently supplied with carbohydrates, the body can convert fat or protein to glucose.

Energy from sugar

Carbohydrate comes in two forms: simple, the sugars, and complex, the starches. Refined sugar (sucrose) is a simple carbohydrate. Whether it is brown or white table sugar, molasses or in a syrup, sucrose provides a quick energy boost. But it provides energy with no nutritional support.

Natural sources of simple sugars (glucose, fructose and maltose) include fruits and milk. These foods offer vital nutrients as well as an immediate supply of energy.

Unlike simple sugars, complex carbohydrates break down slowly in the body and supply their glucose at a steadier rate. And like natural sources of simple sugars, complex carbohydrate foods provide vitamins, minerals and fibre (see p. 46). Popular sources of complex carbohydrates include wholemeal breads, wholewheat pasta, brown rice and potatoes.

Energy from caffeine

A cup of coffee or tea is a widely used antidote to the somnolent effects of a heavy meal. There is proof, at least with coffee drinking, that this self-prescribed antidote to the sleep-inducing effects of food actually works. Tests conducted by psychologists at the University of Wales College, Cardiff, on 32 men and women found that coffee did indeed counteract the after-meal lethargy by boosting alertness. (See also page 82.)

Considering that caffeine is a powerful stimulant mentally and physically (see box, below), this is hardly surprising. New research suggests that caffeine's energising properties are due to its chemical resemblance to a biochemical – adenosine – that

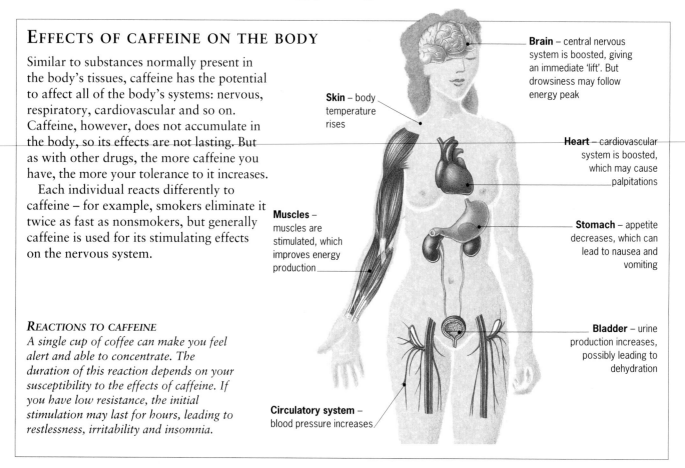

EFFECTS OF CAFFEINE ON THE BODY

Similar to substances normally present in the body's tissues, caffeine has the potential to affect all of the body's systems: nervous, respiratory, cardiovascular and so on. Caffeine, however, does not accumulate in the body, so its effects are not lasting. But as with other drugs, the more caffeine you have, the more your tolerance to it increases.

Each individual reacts differently to caffeine – for example, smokers eliminate it twice as fast as nonsmokers, but generally caffeine is used for its stimulating effects on the nervous system.

REACTIONS TO CAFFEINE
A single cup of coffee can make you feel alert and able to concentrate. The duration of this reaction depends on your susceptibility to the effects of caffeine. If you have low resistance, the initial stimulation may last for hours, leading to restlessness, irritability and insomnia.

Brain – central nervous system is boosted, giving an immediate 'lift'. But drowsiness may follow energy peak

Skin – body temperature rises

Heart – cardiovascular system is boosted, which may cause palpitations

Muscles – muscles are stimulated, which improves energy production

Stomach – appetite decreases, which can lead to nausea and vomiting

Bladder – urine production increases, possibly leading to dehydration

Circulatory system – blood pressure increases

calms some of the brain's activity when it is secreted there. If caffeine is present, your brain's receptor sites will choose it rather than the adenosine and you will remain in a state of alertness.

Other researchers claim that caffeine is only effective as a booster in the short-term, much like a stimulant drug. They say that the initial burst of 'energy' quickly dissipates, leaving the muscles tired.

Natural energisers

Another brain energiser is a naturally occurring compound called choline. A component of acetylcholine, a neurotransmitter, choline may help to relieve some neurological and psychiatric illnesses. Research undertaken by Dr Richard J. Wurtman, a neuroscientist of the Massachusetts Institute of Technology, Cambridge, on Alzheimer's disease suggests that increased levels of choline can enhance memory and revitalise brain cells. Although choline is not a cure, adequate levels of it may help in preventing the disease and further research is under way.

Choline occurs in foods rich in lecithin – egg yolks, meat and fish. Other sources of lecithin include sunflower seeds and foods made from soya beans, such as tofu. Granulated lecithin, available in health food shops, can be used as a dietary supplement.

THE STONE AGE DIET

Since the modern diet of refined carbohydrates and plentiful fat is associated with many maladies, some people have gone back to the Stone Age – in dietary terms. The popular image of prehistoric humans is of successful hunters who feasted on freshly killed meat. But hunting was difficult, dangerous and not always successful – so many of the foods our ancient ancestors depended on were nuts, fruits, roots and vegetables gathered from the wild.

A study of 58 modern hunter-gatherer societies found that about two-thirds of them rely on plants rather than animals for their food. Research by A.S. Truswell, of the University of Sydney, on the !Kung tribe of South Africa revealed a generally healthy group of people whose diet was about 80 per cent vegetarian. They did not exhibit the harmful effects associated with a Western diet, such as obesity, high blood pressure and heart disease.

Adopting a simple diet

Advocates of the Stone Age diet recommend eating more nuts, seeds and berries. They say that the distinctive ingredients of the contemporary diet – such as refined grain and dairy produce, along with coffee, tea, alcohol, tobacco and refined sugars, are the cause of most degenerative Western diseases, as well as many allergies. They are not, however, suggesting that nuts, seeds and berries should be the only foods eaten. A balanced, healthy diet would be impossible with such a limited choice. The idea behind the Stone Age diet is to adopt it for a short time until the body cleanses itself, then to reintroduce other foods one by one while keeping watch for any allergic reactions. However, this should only be done with the help of a nutritionist. Of course, not everyone wants to return to the Stone Age, but that is no reason to miss out on the benefits that these 'original' foods offer.

CHOOSING AND STORING NUTS

Nuts add variety, texture, and nutritional value to sweet and savoury dishes. Here are some tips for getting the best from them.

▶ *To be sure of freshness, always buy from a shop with a high turnover.*

▶ *Where possible, buy nuts in their shells – shelled nuts become rancid quickly because of their high fat content.*

▶ *Avoid shells with cracks, holes or signs of mould.*

▶ *If a nut rattles in its shell it is probably old (except for peanuts – which are not actually nuts but pulses).*

▶ *Store nuts in the refrigerator or in airtight jars in a cool, dry place.*

FOODS OF AN EARLIER AGE

Nuts and seeds are portable, tasty and great energy sources because of their high-fat content including omega-3 fatty acids. In addition to protein (10 to 25 per cent by weight), they offer B vitamins; vitamin E; the minerals iron, calcium, potassium and magnesium; and fibre – all of which are essential for good health.

Berries are also very nutritious. They are a good source of vitamin C, and some, like raspberries and blackberries, are high in fibre. Others have certain medicinal properties.

Nuts and seeds have a high fat content. The fat is mostly unsaturated and is not believed to contribute to atherosclerosis

Cranberries have strong antibiotic and antiviral properties

Raspberries contain natural salicylates, which have anti-inflammatory properties

Strawberries contain natural antioxidants

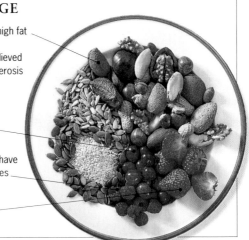

Fighting Infection with

Yoghurt

An ancient food, yoghurt has had many great claims made about its healing properties. It is a valuable source of nutrients and it has the extra bonus of being an excellent infection fighter. Yoghurt is also very easy to make.

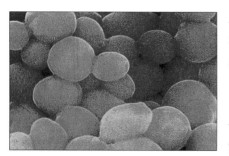

CANDIDA ALBICANS
The yeast candida albicans *causes painful infections. If you are prone to yeast infections, eat 225 g (8 oz) of 'live' yoghurt a day. Yoghurt can also be applied directly to the infected area to bring relief from itching and to help to cure the condition.*

VERSATILE FOOD
Because the milk sugar (lactose) has been broken down by bacteria, yoghurt is more easily digested than milk. This makes it an excellent food for newly weaned babies, elderly people and people suffering from lactose intolerance.

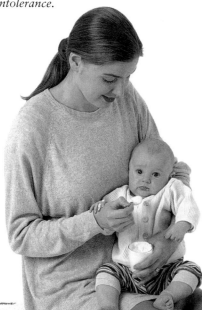

Whatever its healing properties, yoghurt is a nutritional boon. It is a good source of milk nutrients, such as protein, calcium, potassium and riboflavin. Yoghurt is recommended by many medical practitioners to postmenopausal women because it is such a rich source of calcium, which creates bone density, and helps to prevent the brittle-bone disease osteoporosis.

INFECTION-FIGHTING PROPERTIES

Research conducted at the Long Island Jewish Medical Center, New York, has substantiated the claim that yoghurt is an effective treatment for vaginal yeast infections such as thrush. A group of women with a history of chronic yeast infections agreed to eat 225 grams (8 ounces) of 'live' yoghurt containing the *Lactobacillus acidophilus* culture each day for six months. As a result, they suffered far fewer yeast infections than a control group who did not eat yoghurt.

Research by Dr George M. Halpern at the University of California School of Medicine at Davis found that yoghurt may also boost the immune system. People who ate two 225 gram (8 ounce) pots of 'live' yoghurt containing *Lactobacillus bulgaricus* each day for four months had significantly higher blood levels of gamma-interferon, one of the body's infection-fighting substances. Further studies by Dr Halpern found that consuming regular doses of yoghurt also cut

the chances of catching a cold by about 25 per cent, and reduced the symptoms of hay fever by a similar amount. Yoghurt is also thought to increase the activity of NK (natural killer) cells in the body, which attack viruses.

Does only 'live' yoghurt work?
It was previously believed that only yoghurt which contained live cultures of *Lactobacillus bulgaricus*, *Lactobacillus acidophilus* and *Streptococcus thermophilus* had disease-fighting powers. But research by Dr Joseph A. Scimeca at Kraft General Foods in the United States has shown that even yoghurt that has had the majority of its live cultures killed by heating or freezing will still boost the immune system.

THRUSH

A common infection, thrush is caused by the yeast *Candida albicans*. Although it is always present in the body, certain conditions and doses of antibiotics, can cause the yeast to proliferate and produce the infection. Thrush usually affects the vagina but may also affect the mouth, throat and anal area. Vaginal thrush produces a thick white or yellow discharge and intense irritation; oral thrush causes white patches in the mouth; and anal thrush is associated with a rash and irritation.

MAKING YOUR OWN YOGHURT

Yoghurt is cheap and very easy to make. All you need is a saucepan, a thermometer, a bowl or a vacuum flask, 570 ml (1 pint) of milk (any sort will do) and a tablespoon of 'live' plain yoghurt (see opposite).

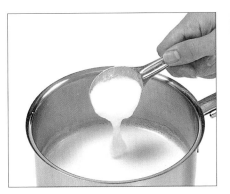

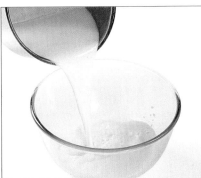

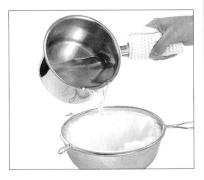

1 *Pour the milk into a saucepan and heat to boiling point. Remove the pan from the heat and allow the milk to cool to 49°C (120°F). Add 1 tablespoon of live plain yoghurt to the milk as a 'starter' and mix thoroughly.*

2 *Pour the mixture into a bowl and cover it with non-PVC cling film. Alternatively, pour the yoghurt mixture into a vacuum flask and then screw down the stopper.*

THICKER TEXTURE
To make a thick Greek-style yoghurt, line a large colander or sieve with gauze or muslin. Pour boiling water through the gauze to scald it. Place the colander or sieve over a bowl, pour in the yoghurt and let it drip overnight.

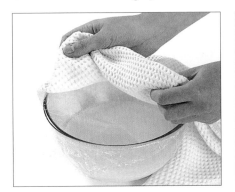

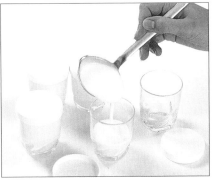

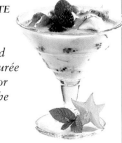

SWEETER TASTE
Add honey, chopped fruit, or unsweetened cooked fruit purée for sweetness or flavour after the yoghurt has been made.

3 *If you are using a bowl, wrap it in a towel and put it in a warm place. Leave the mixture undisturbed until it thickens, usually after eight hours. Be careful not to let the mixture incubate for too long as it may start to separate.*

4 *Pour into pots and eat immediately or refrigerate. Yoghurt will keep for up to five days. Save 1-2 tablespoons of your yoghurt as a 'starter' for the next batch. You may have to buy a fresh 'starter' after making a few batches.*

ICED DESSERT
Frozen yoghurt made with low-fat milk provides a less fattening dessert than ice cream.

IDEAS FOR USING YOGHURT

Yoghurt is delicious eaten on its own, but combining it with other foods can provide a variety of nutritious snacks or meals. Choose low-fat varieties.

▶ *Add yoghurt to soups or casseroles to thicken and add creaminess. When cooking with yoghurt, use a low heat; high temperatures can make the mixture curdle.*

▶ *Use yoghurt as a tasty topping for muesli or fruit desserts, potato salad, baked potatoes and cold pasta dishes.*

▶ *Add lemon rind and paprika to yoghurt to make a sauce for kebabs.*

▶ *Mix fresh herbs and garlic with yoghurt to transform it into a delicious dip or dressing for salads.*

▶ *Use yoghurt instead of cream in cake fillings and toppings.*

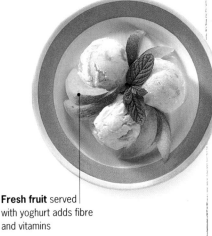

Fresh fruit served with yoghurt adds fibre and vitamins

HARMFUL FOODS?

Not all foods that look and taste appealing are necessarily good for you. Some may cause health risks, while others lead to allergic reactions.

There are a variety of foods that are satisfying and convenient but should only form a small part of a healthy diet. Some people eat fast foods because they have limited time for preparing meals, but in doing so they may be consuming too many unhealthy substances.

Fast food became available on a large scale with the hamburger. It was cheap, instant, filling and very popular. Eventually, a range of other foods – hot dogs, fried chicken, pizzas, kebabs and Chinese and Indian take-aways – became widely available. Although they may not appear to be similar, fast foods have much in common. They tend to be high in calories, fat and salt and low in fibre and some nutrients.

The calories in fast food add up very quickly. A typical meal may contain more than half of your daily calorie needs. Even a beanburger with bun and chips – a favourite with vegetarians – weighs in at a hefty 926 calories, which represents nearly half the daily calorie needs of a typical woman. A very active person might easily burn off these calories, but a more sedentary person would soon find the pounds piling on, perhaps leading to obesity and its associated health problems.

WHAT'S IN A FAST FOOD MEAL?

A typical fast food meal of a cheeseburger, chips and a milk shake provides around 1000 calories, with 17 per cent of the calories coming from protein, 39 per cent from fat and 44 per cent from carbohydrate. In addition, such a meal would contain over 1 000 milligrams of sodium and very little fibre. Many other fast foods are even worse. For instance, a British survey of fast foods found a sweet-and-sour dish from a Chinese takeaway that contained a staggering 2052 calories and 113 grams of fat (1017 calories) per portion. And, since in Britain, fast food outlets are not required by law to disclose what goes into products, the consumer would be blissfully unaware.

The drinks and desserts served in fast food restaurants are often high in sugar. A typical milk shake may contain between 8 and 14 teaspoons of sugar. A 225 millilitre (8 fluid ounce) soft drink contains the equivalent of about five teaspoons of sugar, while a 350 millilitre (12 fluid ounce) drink contains about eight teaspoons.

Fat and fibre

One thing fast food is not short on is fat. Calories derived from fat can range from 30 per cent for a hamburger to 75 per cent for a sausage. A minimum of 20 per cent of the fat used in fast food preparation is saturated because it comes from meat. And even if the additional fat used for frying is unsaturated, it can more than double the caloric value of fast foods. Also, full-fat milk is often used for milkshakes. Too much saturated fat in the diet has been associated with increased levels of cholesterol in the blood, which increase the risk of heart disease.

Fibre, on the other hand, is conspicuous by its very low levels in fast food. The best fibre providers tend to be just those foods not included on a fast food menu – fruits, salads and wholemeal rolls. Furthermore, the buns for burgers and hot dogs are usually made with refined flour. Diets low in fibre can cause constipation and may contribute to the development of colon cancer.

Sodium content

Hamburgers contain about 400 milligrams of sodium and fried chicken servings can have more than 2000 milligrams. Naturally, these figures go even higher if you add salt from a shaker. The biological need for sodium is only about 220 milligrams a day, the equivalent of one-tenth of a teaspoon of

FAST FOOD MEALS

Fast food meals are often popular with many members of the family, but instead of buying takeaways, try making your own quick meals. A homemade version of hamburger and chips is just as tasty and has less fat. Make the burgers from lean minced beef, then grill or bake them. Cut scrubbed, unpeeled potatoes into very thin slices, toss with a spoonful of olive oil, and bake in a hot oven until crisp and golden.

COMMERCIAL FAST FOOD MEAL
A single meal of hamburger, chips, a fizzy orange drink and apple pie from a fast food outlet will provide you with many of the essential nutrients. But the proportions of these nutrients may not be healthy.

A regular portion of chips
provides 268 calories; 3.2 g of protein; 31.2 g of carbohydrate; 14.3 g of fat, of which 3.1 g is saturated; 5.8 g of fibre; and 1000 mg of sodium

A ¼ lb hamburger
provides 244 calories; 13.9 g of protein; 27.7 g of carbohydrate; 8.6 g of fat, of which 4 g is saturated; 2.7 g of fibre; and 400 mg of sodium

A regular fizzy orange drink
provides 83 calories; 22.5 g of carbohydrate (all sugar); and a trace of sodium

An apple pie
provides 219 calories; 2.4 g of protein; 21.4 g of carbohydrate, of which 9.9 g is sugar; 13.8 g of fat, of which 4.5 g is saturated; 4.3 g of fibre; and 200 mg of sodium

salt. The suggested maximum daily sodium intake is somewhat higher – 1100 to 3300 milligrams, however, a fast food diet can quickly exceed these amounts.

The possible harmful effects of excess salt in the diet are well documented, albeit with some controversy. Even though some researchers have linked hypertension (high blood pressure) with a high sodium intake, there is no conclusive proof that sodium can cause it. Eating less salt, however, does help to lower blood pressure.

An unhealthy choice

Although the occasional fast food meal in an otherwise healthy diet will do no harm, a diet overreliant on such convenience foods lacks many of the nutrients and health boosters that are found in fruit and vegetables. It is also distinctly lacking in variety, which is an important feature of a nutritionally balanced diet.

Adolescents, who have high energy requirements, may quickly burn up the calories supplied by fast foods, but these extra calories soon turn to body fat in adults. Eaten regularly, the high-fat, high-salt and low-fibre content of fast foods may lead to serious health problems.

FOOD ADDITIVES

As the popularity of processed foods increases, so does the concern about what manufacturers add to foods. Preservatives

are the most common additive. They are added to food to prevent the growth of dangerous microorganisms, such as bacteria, that can cause food poisoning. Additives are also used to extend the food's shelf life and help to make food much cheaper and more widely available.

All additives in foods that have passed the European Community's safety tests are given an E number. Additives without E numbers are allowed in the United Kingdom but must be mentioned on food labels.

Preservatives

Some of the traditional additives, such as nitrates that are used to cure meats, have been linked with cancer. However, they do prevent botulism, which is a deadly disease.

The benzoate preservatives (E210–219), particularly calcium benzoate (E213), are used for fruit preservation and are found in products like fruit drinks and fruit pies. Some individuals may be sensitive or allergic to these additives. Sulphites (E220–E227) are used to preserve fruits, vegetables and fish, as well as wine, beer and cider. Sulphites should be avoided by asthmatics as they may aggravate asthma attacks.

Antioxidants are added to oils and fats to prevent their reacting with oxygen and turning rancid. Two of these antioxidants, BHA (E320) and BHT (E321), have caused concern. While some studies have shown that BHT acts as a cancer promoter in rats,

TREATING YOUR CHILD
Eating fast food is considered a treat by many children. It may be difficult to wean your children off such foods, but there are ways you can limit their intake. Satisfy a child's appetite with homemade 'fun' foods such as pizzas. Let her add the topping of her choice.

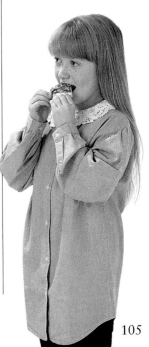

other studies have indicated that it may actually guard against certain cancers, and that rats fed BHT live longer.

Colourings

Dyes are added to food to make it look more appealing to the consumer. These dyes have been highly criticised by consumers because, unlike preservatives, they do not increase the safety of food only 'prettify' it.

Some colourings are natural, but over half of the permitted colourings in the United Kingdom are made in the laboratory. Of these, the most concern has been over the azo, or coal-tar, dyes.

Tartrazine, a yellow azo dye that is often used in children's drinks and sweets, causes allergic reactions in some people. Asthmatics and people who are sensitive to aspirin are more likely to be sensitive to tartrazine

THE PROS AND CONS OF ADDITIVES

If a food contains additives, they should be clearly listed on the label, but the bewildering array of chemical names and numbers may be more confusing than helpful. The chart below describes the types of

additives, the foods that usually contain them, and their positive and negative effects. Use the chart as a guide before shopping to help you make healthier choices. (Also see opposite.)

ADDITIVE	FOOD	PROS	CONS
PRESERVATIVES			
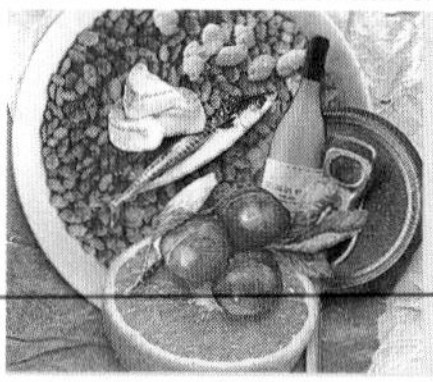 Nitrates, nitrites, BHT, BHA, benzoic acid, benzoates, ascorbic acid, sulphites.	Nitrates in vegetables; nitrites in cured meats; BHT and BHA in margarine and crisps; benzoates in fruit drinks; sulphites in fruit juice, beer, wine and cider.	Protect food from bacteria and fungi, protecting against food poisoning. Extend shelf life.	Nitrites are linked with cancer. Sulphites and benzoates can cause adverse reactions in asthmatics.
COLOURINGS			
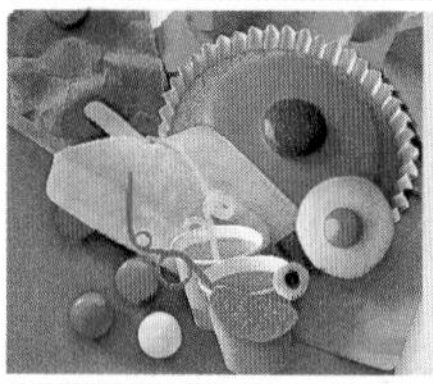 Natural substances, such as beta carotene. Tartrazine and other azo, or cold-tar, dyes.	Majority of processed foods. Tartrazine in children's drinks and sweets.	Make food look more appetising.	Azo dyes can cause allergic reaction in asthmatics.
FLAVOUR ENHANCERS			
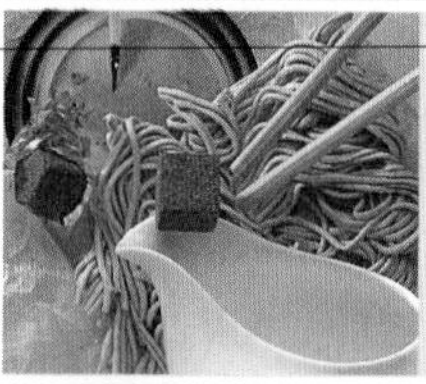 Monosodium glutamate, hydrolysed vegetable protein.	Chinese food, gravy, soups and snacks.	Enhance flavour.	Allegedly cause allergic reactions in some people.
STABILISERS AND THICKENERS			
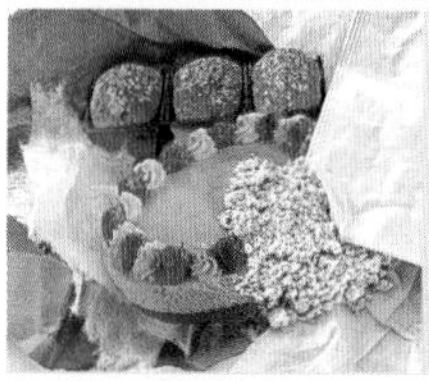 Gums, pectin, gelatine, cellulose, seaweeds.	Processed desserts, sauces, soups and baked foods.	Improve consistency and texture.	Make food look more substantial than it really is. Large amounts can cause flatulence.
EMULSIFIERS			
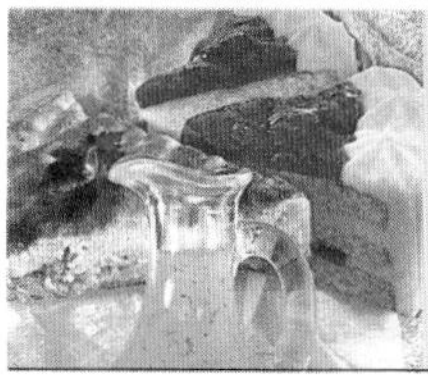 Lecithin, acacia.	Baked food, frozen puddings and dressings.	Stop oil and water particles from separating.	Acacia causes allergic reactions in some people.

Chinese restaurant syndrome

In 1968, half an hour after beginning to eat a meal in a Chinese restaurant, an American physician suffered extreme discomfort. His head ached and he felt a burning sensation in the back of his neck. The symptoms were traced to a high ingestion of monosodium glutamate (MSG), a flavour enhancer often used in Chinese cooking. The doctor later called this the Chinese Restaurant Syndrome. Many other people claimed they had similar experiences after eating Chinese food. The latest evidence, however, has shown that MSG is innocent. Other constituents of Chinese food, such as shellfish and fermented soya sauce, are suspected of causing Chinese Restaurant Syndrome.

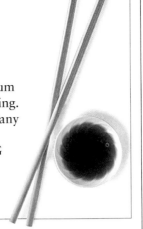

and other azo dyes. There is worldwide concern over coal-tar food dyes but little unanimity. Sixteen are permitted in the United Kingdom, but only five are allowed in the United States. Tartrazine is banned in France and Belgium. The coal-tar dye, red dye number 2, is banned in the United States, whereas it is permitted in Canada, which bans red dye number 40. Norway has gone one step further by putting a blanket ban on all 'artificial' food colourings.

Flavourings

Thousands of different flavourings are added to processed foods. Some are natural, others are synthetic copies of natural substances. Neither the natural flavourings nor their synthetics are thought to be a problem. But monosodium glutamate (or MSG E621), which strictly speaking is a flavour enhancer, is alleged to cause adverse reactions in some people. It is added to many savoury foods, soups and Chinese food – hence the nickname Chinese Restaurant Syndrome to describe its possible effects in sensitive people (see box, above).

MSG is present naturally in tomatoes, anchovies and Parmesan cheese, which is why they enhance flavours of other foods.

Thickeners and emulsifiers

Thickening or bulking agents increase the amount of air or water a product can hold. Derived from natural substances like seaweed and vegetable celluloses, these are generally harmless but large amounts of some thickeners may cause abdominal distension.

Emulsifiers prevent the oil and water from separating in processed foods like mayonnaise. Lecithin, derived from soya bean sources, is a popular emulsifier. It is natural

and considered harmless. There have been reports, however, that the emulsifier acacia, which is found in frozen puddings and baked foods, causes an allergic reaction in some people.

FOOD ALLERGIES AND INTOLERANCES

It is not only spoiled food and additives that can make people ill. Allergies or intolerances to many foods are widespread and seem to be increasing. A true food allergy, as opposed to an intolerance, provokes an abnormal response from the immune system. Compounds in usually harmless foods are mistaken for alien invaders by the immune system, which responds by launching antibodies to combat the threat. The antibodies cause the release of powerful inflammatory substances that can provoke a range of symptoms, from diarrhoea and nausea to a potentially fatal swelling of the throat. Allergic symptoms usually manifest themselves in minutes, thus alerting susceptible people immediately to the problematic foods. Foods most likely to provoke reactions are milk, eggs, wheat, fish, shellfish, strawberries, nuts and pulses, especially soya beans and peanuts. Unless the allergy disappears of its own accord, usually the only recourse is to cut the offending food out of the diet.

What is food intolerance?

True food allergies are rare, but food intolerances are fairly common. The adverse reactions can take hours or even days to set in because, unlike the case with true allergies, the immune system is not affected by food intolerance. Symptoms range from mild maladies like headaches, indigestion,

TAKING PRECAUTIONS

Protecting yourself from the potential hazards of some food additives is quite simple if you follow these suggestions:

▶ *Eat fresh or minimally processed foods. The more natural a form the food is in, the fewer additives it is likely to contain.*

▶ *Eat a wide variety of foods. This will minimise the chances of any one additive reaching a 'dangerous' level in your body.*

▶ *Eat 'real food' not the artificial equivalent. For example, fresh or frozen orange juice is preferable to artificially flavoured, coloured and sweetened fruit drinks.*

▶ *Avoid fast foods if possible, or eat them sparingly.*

▶ *Read the food labels. Most additives are listed but not all. Select the ones that have the least artificial additives.*

▶ *Make a list of additives you are concerned about and take it with you when you go shopping.*

Food diary

If you think you may be suffering from an intolerance to something in your diet, keep a record of what you eat and whether or not you have any adverse reactions afterwards. This will help you to detect problem foods as a pattern of illness may emerge.

Note the date, time, and all the food and drink consumed. It often takes many hours for particular reactions to occur, so fill in your diary over several days or weeks. (See also page 14.)

depression and diarrhoea to chronic conditions such as rheumatoid arthritis, eczema and irritable bowel syndrome.

According to a study by Dr John O. Hunter of Addenbrookes Hospital in Cambridge, in 1982, cereals, dairy products, products containing caffeine, yeast-based items and citrus fruits are the most common sources of food intolerance. Wheat is the most troublesome food, upsetting 60 per cent of trial subjects.

Enzyme deficiency

Two common food intolerances are known to be the result of an enzyme deficiency. Lactose intolerance is very common, especially among people of Asian, African or Mediterranean descent. These people lack an enzyme in their intestine called lactase without which the lactose (milk sugar) in milk and dairy products, such as butter and cheese, cannot be broken down, resulting in symptoms such as stomach cramps, diarrhoea and gas. Similarly, a deficiency of the

enzyme lipase in the intestine can result in problems with fats passing undigested into the lower part of the bowel.

Identifying the guilty foods

Food intolerance is often difficult to diagnose. Special clinics for treating food intolerance and allergy, which have proliferated in recent years, use a number of different methods to identify troublesome foods.

In patch tests, food samples are placed on the skin to see if an allergic reaction takes place. But the same allergic reaction may not occur internally when the food is eaten. Another method, the elimination diet, banishes all but a few innocuous foods from the diet for a few days. Foods are then reintroduced one by one while any reactions are noted. But this method may not be entirely reliable because the patient's expectations of a bad reaction to a particular food could trigger psycho-somatic illness.

Double-blind trials are probably the best way of identifying food reactions. Food suspected of causing a reaction is put into a capsule, while an identical capsule is filled with a nonreactive substance. Neither the doctor nor the patient knows which capsule contains the food. The patient then swallows one of the capsules and records whether or not it triggers a reaction. A true reaction will only occur when a capsule with food in it is swallowed. Providing that the offending food can be identified, cutting it out of the diet is an effective treatment.

Cutting out gluten

Once it is known that a food causes a reaction, the obvious treatment is to stop eating it. But, as many people who cannot eat wheat products have found, this is not always as simple as it sounds.

People with an intolerance to wheat are actually reacting to gluten, a protein found not only in wheat but in rye, oats and barley. If gluten is eaten by people who are intolerant to it, they suffer from abdominal pains and diarrhoea. Even the tiny amount of gluten in a communion wafer can trigger irritation in some individuals.

In rare cases, the gluten intolerance is part of a disorder called coeliac disease in which a person is unable to absorb essential nutrients from the intestines. The condition may lead to other health problems, such as anaemia. If you think you or your child

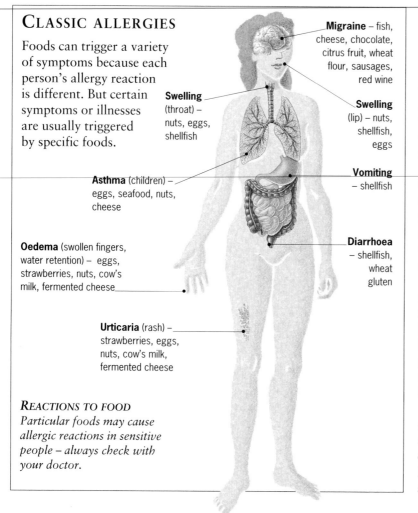

CLASSIC ALLERGIES

Foods can trigger a variety of symptoms because each person's allergy reaction is different. But certain symptoms or illnesses are usually triggered by specific foods.

Swelling (throat) – nuts, eggs, shellfish

Asthma (children) – eggs, seafood, nuts, cheese

Oedema (swollen fingers, water retention) – eggs, strawberries, nuts, cow's milk, fermented cheese

Urticaria (rash) – strawberries, eggs, nuts, cow's milk, fermented cheese

Migraine – fish, cheese, chocolate, citrus fruit, wheat flour, sausages, red wine

Swelling (lip) – nuts, shellfish, eggs

Vomiting – shellfish

Diarrhoea – shellfish, wheat gluten

REACTIONS TO FOOD
Particular foods may cause allergic reactions in sensitive people – always check with your doctor.

suffer from gluten intolerance, it is essential that you visit the doctor for diagnosis. The disorder cannot be cured, but elimination of gluten from the diet helps to restore the person to normal health.

Identifying an obvious gluten-containing food such as bread is fairly straightforward. Cakes, biscuits, muesli, porridge and pasta are also easy to single out. But problems arise with processed and ready-made foods. Wheat flour is often used as a thickener and is found in all sorts of foods. Food labels can help but may not be foolproof. The following can mean that there is gluten in the food: edible starch, mixed grain, whole grain, multigrain, vegetable protein, food starch, starch, rusk, thickener and bran.

Faced with such a minefield, sufferers often settle for a diet without any processed foods. Dried beans, nuts, rice and corn are used as staples. Eggs, beans, fish, milk, cheese and meat provide protein. Vitamins can be had from fruits and vegetables. And variety can come in the form of butter, cream, herbs, honey, jam, salt, spices, sugars, tea, wine and yoghurt.

THE CHOLESTEROL CONNECTION
A high level of cholesterol in the blood is associated with a narrowing of the arteries (atherosclerosis), hypertension and heart disease. But reducing your cholesterol level need not mean unreasonably restricting your diet. By eating the right foods, you can encourage your body to shed excess cholesterol.

Reducing the amount of high-cholesterol foods like eggs and cheese in your diet does help to reduce the body's cholesterol level, but not enough, because the body makes its own cholesterol. This waxlike substance is essential for many vital processes such as producing new cells and certain hormones. Depending on your body weight, from 800 to 1000 milligrams of cholesterol is produced each day in the liver. The body also operates a balancing mechanism: when extra cholesterol enters the system through diet, less is produced in the body and more is excreted. Thus in most people, the cholesterol level stays much the same all the time.

Is cholesterol harmful?
Although there is little doubt about the relationship between high serum, or blood, cholesterol levels and heart disease, questions arise about the role of dietary cholesterol in heart disease. Many scientists maintain that a diet high in saturated fat (which the liver uses to manufacture cholesterol) is the main cause of high blood cholesterol levels, not foods rich in cholesterol itself, such as eggs, kidneys, liver, cheese and prawns.

Children and food reactions
Genuine allergies are far less common than is generally believed, and although some reactions to food allergies are dangerous, most mild food reactions tend to disappear with age. Some reactions to food, however, are more serious and can affect the absorption of nutrients, leading sometimes to dangerous weight loss or stunted growth. One such condition is coeliac disease. Approximately one child in 2000 suffers from an intolerance to gluten, found in oats, barley, rye and wheat that leads to an inflammation of the small bowel. A gluten-free diet is the only way to relieve the symptoms. Other common food reactions are to milk, tea, eggs, chocolate, soya and corn.

WHAT TRIGGERS AN ALLERGIC REACTION?

When allergens enter the body, they cause a reaction with the mast cells, special cells most commonly found in the linings of the stomach and lungs. These mast cells become covered in specific immunoglobin E (IgE) molecules, which attach themselves to the mast cells as part of the body's defence against invading allergens.

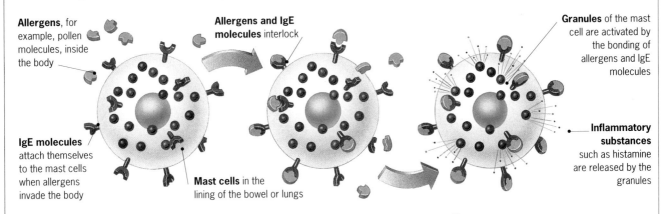

Allergens, for example, pollen molecules, inside the body

Allergens and IgE molecules interlock

Granules of the mast cell are activated by the bonding of allergens and IgE molecules

IgE molecules attach themselves to the mast cells when allergens invade the body

Mast cells in the lining of the bowel or lungs

Inflammatory substances such as histamine are released by the granules

SUSPECT MOLECULES
Allergen molecules enter the body via food, such as the protein in peanuts, or by inhalation, for example, pollen.

INTERLOCKING
The allergen molecules bind with the IgE molecules, which are attached to the mast cells at particular points.

PROVOKING A SYMPTOM
The mast cell granules release inflammatory substances such as histamine, which cause headaches.

In support of this theory, studies at Rockefeller University in New York discovered that an egg-rich diet raised the blood cholesterol levels in only two out of five people. And an analysis by Paul N. Hopkins of the University of Utah in Salt Lake City of various studies on cholesterol concluded that in most people a high-cholesterol diet rarely raises blood cholesterol levels.

Not all research comes to the same conclusion, however. A study by Dr Richard Shekelle, professor of epidemiology at the University of Texas in Houston, found that people who ate high levels of cholesterol-rich foods lived an average of three years less than those with low-cholesterol diets. He also found evidence that a high intake of dietary cholesterol could stimulate the blood to make more clots, which could promote heart disease.

But although these findings seem contradictory, organisations that promote good health, such as the British Heart Foundation, do recommend a reduction in the intake of high-cholesterol foods. Their main recommendation, however, is to cut down on foods containing saturated fats as these fats have a greater effect in pushing up blood cholesterol levels than dietary cholesterol.

WHAT IS 'GOOD' CHOLESTEROL?

Cholesterol is categorised in different types according to how it is linked to the protein carrier: the 'good' or 'helpful' kind is HDL (high-density lipoprotein), and the 'bad' is LDL (low-density lipoprotein). There are also VLDLs (very low-density lipoproteins). High levels of LDLs are associated with clogging of the arteries, which causes heart disease. High levels of HDLs, on the other hand, help to prevent this from happening because they collect and remove excess cholesterol from tissues and serum. Certain foods can reduce LDLs and boost HDLs, thus protecting against heart disease.

Foods that boost HDLs

In 23 out of 25 studies, oat bran has been shown to reduce overall levels of cholesterol. More interesting, though, is the fact that oat bran may reduce detrimental LDLs and boost beneficial HDLs. Researchers have claimed that oatbran boosts HDLs by about 15 per cent after two or three months. Oat bran's weapon against cholesterol is believed to be high levels of beta glucans, a soluble fibre (see p. 46).

The pectin in fresh vegetables and fruits also provides soluble fibre; good choices include brussels sprouts, parsnips, turnips, okra, peas, broccoli, oranges, apricots and mangoes. Research conducted by Dr James Anderson, of the University of Kentucky College of Medicine, revealed that just one cup a day of a food rich in soluble fibre – like oat bran – reduces bad LDLs by about 20 per cent, and boosts good HDLs by nine per cent in the long term.

CLOGGING THE ARTERIES

Heart disease is caused by reduced blood flow to the heart muscle because of narrowed arteries (atherosclerosis). High levels of LDLs ('bad' cholesterol) penetrate the inner lining of the artery and become trapped there.

Macrophages (white blood cells that normally scavenge and inactivate or kill infectious and foreign agents) swallow the LDLs and combine with the platelets (blood cells that assist in blood coagulation) to form plaques. Over the years, these plaques slowly build up, narrowing, and possibly blocking, the artery, making clotting more likely to occur. This will cause complete blockage of the artery.

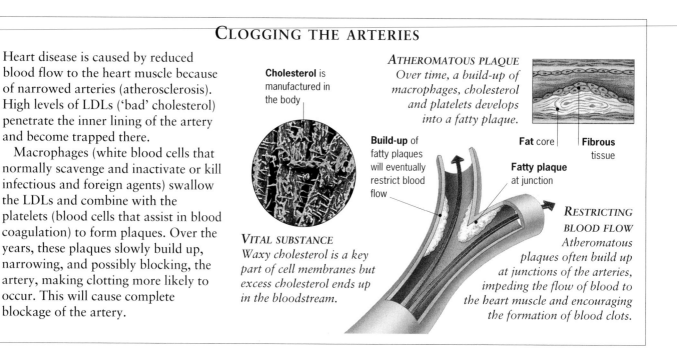

Cholesterol is manufactured in the body

VITAL SUBSTANCE
Waxy cholesterol is a key part of cell membranes but excess cholesterol ends up in the bloodstream.

ATHEROMATOUS PLAQUE
Over time, a build-up of macrophages, cholesterol and platelets develops into a fatty plaque.

Build-up of fatty plaques will eventually restrict blood flow

Fat core

Fibrous tissue

Fatty plaque at junction

RESTRICTING BLOOD FLOW
Atheromatous plaques often build up at junctions of the arteries, impeding the flow of blood to the heart muscle and encouraging the formation of blood clots.

The benefits of alcohol

Drinking alcohol – in moderate amounts – is also credited with protecting the heart from disease. Some researchers point to the puzzling fact that in France the incidence of heart disease is much lower than in the rest of Europe although the French eat a very high-cholesterol diet (see p. 80). Their habit of drinking wine with meals is cited by some researchers as the protective factor. The wine is said to increase HDL cholesterol, thus lowering the risk of heart disease.

Like wine, beer can raise the level of good HDLs. A study in the United Kingdom found that a moderate intake of alcohol – a glass or two a day – boosted HDLs by about seven per cent. A similar study had even better results – boosting HDLs by 17 per cent with a daily intake of 1.3 ounces of alcohol. But experts do not advocate excessive drinking. Alcohol can increase the risk of high blood pressure, which may lead to heart disease.

Cooking oil and cholesterol

It is well known that eating saturated fat stimulates cholesterol synthesis in the body. Polyunsaturated fats, on the other hand, which are found in vegetable oils, have been shown in tests to lower overall cholesterol levels by ten per cent. But better still seems to be the monounsaturated fat in olive and rapeseed oils. This fat not only lowers over-all cholesterol levels, but also raises the level of good HDLs.

How does olive oil help?

Some scientists believe that olive oil protects the heart in a third way. This has to do with the way that LDLs clog the arteries. The theory is that rogue molecules called free radicals collide with the LDLs, becoming fixed to them via an oxygen link. These 'oxidised' LDLs are then swallowed up by macrophages, white blood cells that normally protect against foreign bodies and infectious fungi bacteria or viruses. The macrophages then join up with platelets, making enlarged cells that go on to form fatty plaques that build up over many years, restricting blood flow (see opposite).

Olive oil may protect against this oxidation in two ways. Whereas polyunsaturated fats are readily oxidised, the monounsaturated fat in olive oil is less prone to damage from oxidation. Second, olive oil contains antioxidants, such as vitamin E, that are thought to mop up free radicals, thus reducing the likelihood of LDLs coming under attack in the first place. The role of antioxidants in preventing disease appears to be increasingly influential.

However olive oil works, there is little doubt that it is effective. In Mediterranean countries, such as Italy and Greece, where olive oil is the primary cooking oil, the rates of heart disease are significantly lower than in countries like the United States – despite similar intakes of fat and cholesterol in the diet (see p. 114).

Cholesterol levels

The recommended level of cholesterol for people of any age is under 5.2 millimoles per litre (mmol/l) of blood. If your cholesterol level is over 6.5 mmol/l, your doctor will measure the amount of HDLs and LDLs that are present. But even if your cholesterol is below 5.2 mmol/l, the relative levels of high and low-density lipoproteins is an important factor in determining your risk. Women, particularly premenopausal women, tend to have higher levels of HDLs than men because oestrogen raises the level of HDLs. A level of 1.55 mmol/l or above of HDLs will offer protection against heart disease. The risk of heart disease is increased if the level of HDLs is 0.9 mmol/l or below. A dangerous level of LDLs in cholesterol is 4.1 mmol/l or more; an amount under 3.4 mmol/l is preferred.

'GOOD'-CHOLESTEROL DIET

Eating foods that help to increase 'good' cholesterol (HDL) and reduce overall cholesterol levels does not have to mean a sudden dramatic change to your diet. You will be more likely to maintain a healthy diet if you introduce the following measures gradually.

► *Boost your intake of lean foods, such as fish and lean meat, while reducing fats high in saturates, such as hard margarine products.*

► *Eat porridge for breakfast.*

► *Eat plenty of fresh fruits and vegetables, at least five servings per day.*

► *A moderate amount of alcohol can boost HDL levels. But too much alcohol can have the opposite effect.*

► *Increase your intake of dried beans, grapefruit, bran, garlic, onions, apples, shiitake mushrooms, almonds and walnuts – all may lower overall cholesterol levels.*

LIFE-ENHANCING OIL
Use polyunsaturated fats like corn oil and sunflower oil for cooking or in salads. Better still, use olive or rapeseed oils, which are high in monounsaturates.

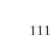

FRESH OR STALE?

Because eggs are highly perishable, special care should be taken to prevent illness. Observe these simple precautions when choosing and storing eggs.

▶ *Always check the sell-by date on cartons.*

▶ *Do not use cracked eggs because they may contain bacteria.*

▶ *Store eggs in the refrigerator, not on a work surface. Store leftover raw eggs in a tightly covered container; they will keep for two days in the refrigerator. Egg whites keep for up to two weeks.*

▶ *Store eggs pointed end downwards.*

▶ *Eat egg dishes at once, or refrigerate them. It is vital that people 'at risk' from salmonella – babies, children, pregnant women and elderly people – should not eat raw eggs at all.*

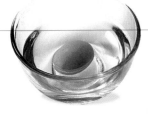

TOO OLD TO USE
To test the freshness of an egg, put it in a bowl of water. Fresh eggs sink to the bottom, while stale eggs float rounded end up, to the top because the size of the air pocket increases with age.

THE TRUTH ABOUT EGGS

Cheap, nutritious and versatile – what could be better than an egg? But scares about cholesterol and salmonella have tarnished its reputation in recent years.

Nutritionally, eggs have much to recommend them. The average egg contains about six grams of very high-quality protein, which is roughly 15 per cent of an adult's daily requirement. An egg also supplies many important vitamins and minerals, including iron, calcium, and vitamins A, B, D and E. It is also low in calories (there are only 75 calories in a large egg).

It is not surprising, then, that eggs were once considered an almost perfect food, and a high consumption was recommended. But unfortunately, research into cholesterol showed that, at about 213 milligrams per large egg, their cholesterol content is high. Since the suggested daily intake of cholesterol is only 300 milligrams, it is easy to see why dietary guidelines now recommend limiting your egg intake to two or three a week. And, to be consistent, you should also limit your intake of other high-cholesterol foods, such as prawns and lobster.

Some farmers in the United States have responded to people's worries over cholesterol by claiming to have produced a 'low cholesterol' egg through selective breeding and cholesterol-lowering feeds, such as fish oil. Even if the eggs are lower in cholesterol, say 175 milligrams against the usual 213, they still pack a cholesterol punch in excess of most foods.

Using less egg yolk

Concerned consumers can reduce their cholesterol intake in better ways. All of an egg's cholesterol (and most of its nutrients) is found in the yolk. The white is mainly protein. In dishes like omelettes two whites can be substituted for one whole egg. In baking, a whole egg can be replaced with two egg whites, and two whole eggs can be replaced with one whole egg plus two or three whites. People who want to reduce cholesterol even more can use egg substitutes. These are frozen or powdered and usually contain very little cholesterol as they are made from egg whites and monounsaturated oils. The main drawback is that egg substitutes also contain artificial additives.

Salmonella

The danger of salmonella poisoning from eggs has received massive publicity in recent years. Many hens harbour the disease-causing bacteria *Salmonella enteritidis*, which can be passed into the egg before the shell is formed. The result is a perfect-looking egg that is contaminated.

The salmonella bacteria can be destroyed by cooking. But some researchers claim that normal cooking temperatures are not high enough to do this. The bacteria could still survive in lightly cooked dishes such as soft-boiled or scrambled eggs, runny omelettes and light soufflés. Uncooked food, like the raw egg in Caesar salad or homemade mayonnaise, is particularly prone to infection.

Salmonella poisoning is especially dangerous for those people whose ability to fight disease may be immature or impaired, children, the elderly and people with chronic illnesses. Pregnant women, too, can risk passing the infection on to their unborn babies. Those at risk should use an egg substitute or liquid pasteurised egg products, which are heat-treated to kill any pathogenic bacteria.

NUTRIENTS IN EGGS

PRODUCT	CALORIES	PROTEIN (grams)	CARBOHYDRATE (grams)	FAT (grams)	CHOLESTEROL (milligrams)	SODIUM (milligrams)
Whole egg (1 large)	75	6.3	0.6	5.1	213	62
Egg yolk (1 large)	59	2.8	0.3	5.1	213	7
Egg white (1 large)	16	3.5	0.3	0	0	55
Egg substitute (30 g/1 oz)	25	3.6	1	0	0	53

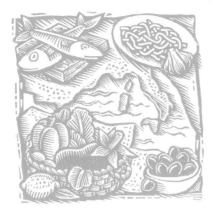

CHAPTER 8

EATING THE BEST DIET

*Some nations are generally
healthier than others and many individuals
might benefit by including in their diets the
nourishing, tasty foods eaten by people in the
regions around the Mediterranean sea, and in Japan
and China. Conspicuously absent from these diets
are the large portions of fatty meats, rich dairy
products, sugary confections and highly refined
and processed foods consumed by urban,
industrialised Western peoples.*

WHAT ARE THE BEST DIETS IN THE WORLD?

Living a long and healthy life depends on a variety of factors, and a well-balanced diet is one of the most vital. This is demonstrated clearly by the different effects of national diets.

A flavour of the Mediterranean
Enhance your meals by experimenting with pulses the Mediterranean way. Add chickpeas, lentils or black-eyed beans to soups and stews. Serve salads of red kidney beans dressed with olive oil, lemon juice, crushed garlic and fresh herbs. Or make dips and spreads by puréeing the beans with the dressing.

Every few years, in the popular press, tales are told of remote, mountainous districts where residents live, hale and hearty, well past their 100th birthdays. The robust health and enviable energy of these individuals are attributed to some special ingredient found in the local diet. The elixir may be live yoghurt, wild garlic or a particular sort of honey, but the claims made for it are sufficient to create a significant sales boom among health-conscious consumers.

Although no one has yet found the recipe for immortality, more than half a century of scientific research has indicated that there are indeed parts of the world where the inhabitants enjoy lives that are far healthier than those of other regions. According to these studies, the traditional diets of the Chinese, Japanese and peoples of the regions bordering the Mediterranean Sea provide safeguards against a broad spectrum of debilitating illnesses, ranging from heart disease to a number of different cancers.

A WORLD OF DIFFERENCE
Within Europe itself, nutritionists have observed that a country's diet seems to become healthier in proportion to its proximity

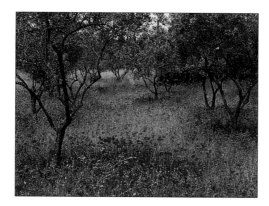

to the Mediterranean Sea. In the 1960s, for instance, a survey of food consumption patterns revealed that the average Spanish and Italian citizen ate more than three times as many fresh fruits and vegetables in a year than his or her counterpart in Great Britain. And although diet may not be the only influence, it seems to be no coincidence that the two countries with the worst rates for cardiovascular disease are Scotland and Finland – both with very low intakes of fruits and vegetables.

It was only in the mid-20th century that links between food and health began to be investigated on a truly scientific basis. The statistics that began to accumulate revealed that even among affluent, developed nations with very similar standards of living, there were dramatic differences in the health of their populations.

Ground-breaking study
In the early 1950s, an American nutritionist, Professor Ancel Keys, launched his ground-breaking 'Seven Countries Study', a detailed scrutiny of the relationship between specific diseases and cultural variations in diet. Keys noted that only a very small proportion of people eating Mediterranean diets, like those of the Italians and Spanish, developed heart disease, in marked contrast to their US counterparts, who were experiencing an increase in such cardiovascular complaints as hypertension, heart attacks and strokes. Working with an international team, Keys established a close connection between dietary fat, blood cholesterol levels and the incidence of heart disease.

For ten years, Keys and his colleagues studied men, aged between 40 and 59 years, who lived in rural areas on three different

FRUIT OF THE OLIVE TREE
Olives are harvested in many Mediterranean lands – Spain, Greece, Italy and Provence in the south of France. Like wine, the oils produced from olives have unique flavours and aromas that are dependent on the country of origin.

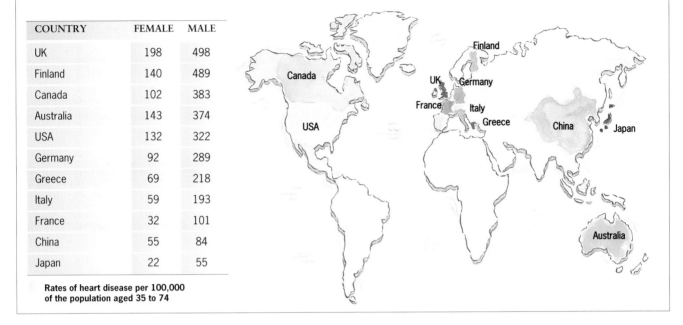

RATES OF HEART DISEASE AROUND THE WORLD

Studies comparing the mortality rates from heart disease have shown marked contrasts between people eating different diets. People who eat a diet high in saturated fats but low in polyunsaturated fats, fruits and vegetables, have a greater risk of developing heart disease than people with healthier diets.

COUNTRY	FEMALE	MALE
UK	198	498
Finland	140	489
Canada	102	383
Australia	143	374
USA	132	322
Germany	92	289
Greece	69	218
Italy	59	193
France	32	101
China	55	84
Japan	22	55

Rates of heart disease per 100,000 of the population aged 35 to 74

continents in seven different countries: the United States, Finland, Italy, Yugoslavia, the Netherlands, Greece and Japan. A systematic comparison of these regional diets revealed that in places where a lot of foods containing large amounts of hard (saturated) fats from animal sources were eaten there were also higher levels of blood cholesterol. These populations also had a greater risk of dying of heart disease. But this higher death rate did not seem to be linked to the total amount of fat in the diet nor to the number of calories eaten.

THE PROTECTIVE OILS

Researchers found the incidence of heart disease to be substantially lower among those subjects eating diets rich in polyunsaturated fats, the fats found in vegetable oils, or in monounsaturated fats, the fats found in olive oil. The Mediterranean diet, in particular, with its lavish use of olive oil, seemed to have a protective effect. Later research into the complicated subject of blood (serum) cholesterol has confirmed this view. The monounsaturated fats found in olive oil appear to lower the total quantity of cholesterol and the dangerous type of cholesterol (known as LDL) that clogs the arteries, while at the same time increasing

the amount of protective cholesterol (HDL) within the bloodstream, which clears excess cholesterol from the blood (see p. 56).

More recent studies have reinforced the merits of the Mediterranean approach to food. The French National Institute for Health and Medical Research in Lyons set up a controlled experiment for two groups of heart-attack patients. In this study, one set of subjects followed a Mediterranean-style diet using rapeseed oil, which is rich in omega-3 fatty acids. The researchers used the other team as a control group, and let them eat whatever they pleased.

After two years the researchers found that the death rate among the Mediterranean group was 70 per cent lower compared to that among the controls. With such clear evidence, they immediately abandoned the clinical trial and put the surviving members of the control group on the Mediterranean-style diet that they were now convinced would improve many patients' longevity.

MODERN DISEASES

Every traditional diet is subject to change. In many parts of the world, in the second half of the 20th century, living standards have risen, science and technology have advanced dramatically, and people have moved in

The antioxidant effect

The bountiful supply of natural antioxidants, such as vitamins C and E and beta carotene, within the Mediterranean diet provides an armoury of powerful defences. These potent chemicals fight the destructive effects of free radicals and oxidants – rogue molecules that are formed in the body as a result of combining with oxygen and environmental and dietary contaminants (see p. 94).

Lemons, oranges, tomatoes, red peppers, avocados and parsley are all endowed with effective natural antioxidants.

MAKING YOUR OWN PASTA

Pasta is an extremely versatile food and a good source of carbohydrate, which provides a steady supply of energy. It is simple to make; the only ingredients you need are 3 eggs and 280 grams (10 ounces) of flour. Let the noodles dry and then cook them in plenty of boiling, lightly salted water.

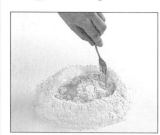

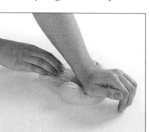

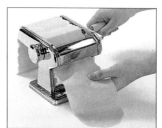

4 Cut the rolled-out pasta into strips about 30 cm (12 in) long. Pass the strips through the cutting rollers of the machine. Support the noodles with your hand.

1 Pour the flour into a mound on a smooth work surface. Make a well in the centre and add the beaten eggs. Draw the flour into the eggs.

2 Hold the dough with one hand and use the heel of your other hand to push the dough away from you. Repeat, rotating the dough, until smooth.

3 Feed a portion of lightly rolled-out dough through a pasta machine. Guide the dough through, taking care not to stretch or pull it.

The value of garlic
Garlic performs a number of healthy functions in the body. It is said to reduce the risk of heart disease by decreasing total blood cholesterol. Also, new research at Pennsylvania State University reveals that a compound in garlic, diallyl disulfide (DAS), depresses the growth of colon, lung and skin cancer cells.

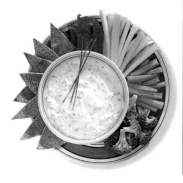

*ENJOYING GARLIC RAW
Raw garlic's pungent flavour can be partially disguised in a yoghurt and herb dip.*

massive numbers from the countryside into ever-expanding cities. But this modernisation has had its drawbacks. As the incidence of traditional infectious diseases decreased, people fell prey to what were, for them, a new set of plagues – illnesses linked with the lifestyles of the industrialised world.

For epidemiologists (scientists who deal with the causes and distribution of diseases affecting a population), the link between Westernisation and the onset of particular diseases became easy to predict. As a country became more industrialised and more affluent, as its rural peasants turned into urban workers and their diets changed, the mortality rates from ailments such as heart disease and diabetes rose.

Ironically, it was these changes in eating habits and their demonstrated injurious effect on the public's health, that proved the value of the now-threatened traditional diets. In Greece, for instance, Professor Antonia Trichopoulou, of the National School of Public Health, monitored the effects on the nation's well-being as people began to abandon the healthy diet that had sustained their ancestors for thousands of years. In 1989 she published a study showing that a dramatic rise in mortality rates from heart disease, diabetes, and cancers of the breast and colon had gone hand in hand with a 20-year increase in the consumption of animal fats and a corresponding decline in fruit and vegetable consumption. Now Greece, in

common with many other Mediterranean countries, is enthusiastically urging its citizens to return to the culinary traditions that nourished their great-grandparents.

A FEAST OF HEALTH
Anyone who takes pleasure in the vibrant colours and flavours of fresh fruits and vegetables, who savours the richness of good olive oil, the tang of lemon juice and the aromas of fresh herbs and garlic, will find no difficulty in embracing a Mediterranean-style diet. Much of it is familiar to lovers of good food: hearty vegetable and bean soups, a generous helping of pasta lightly sauced with tomatoes and basil, a salad bowl full of crisp green leaves tossed with an olive oil dressing, and the freshest possible fish are all hallmarks of Mediterranean cuisine. A culinary voyage from Spain to southern France and Italy and on to Greece would reveal that, while different herbs or flavourings prevail, the general principles remain the same.

These dishes are endowed with elements that promote good health. The dark-fleshed, oily fish beloved by Mediterranean diners – tuna, mackerel, sardines and many other varieties – are rich in omega-3 fatty acids. The unsaturated fats in these fish are also believed to have a strong protective effect on the heart and the entire vascular system, as well as to act as a deterrent against certain types of cancer and other diseases.

The Mediterranean lands abound with grains, vegetables and fruits that thrive in their fertile soils. Incorporated into the diet, these foods provide dietary fibre – another essential ingredient for a truly healthy diet.

ORIENTAL DELIGHTS

Half a world away from the olive groves and vineyards of the Mediterranean shores, the traditional cooks of Japan and China have their own repertoire of life-enhancing, health-preserving foods and culinary techniques. The international scientific community has shown particular interest in the Japanese diet since the citizens of Japan enjoy the world's highest life expectancy and the lowest incidence of heart disease and breast cancer. They do, however, suffer from a high rate of stomach cancer, which is thought to be linked to their heavy consumption of salty, pickled foods.

To a Japanese of traditional tastes, a meal centres upon complex carbohydrates, which are usually provided by several bowlfuls of rice. To vary the menu, Japanese cooks turn to a variety of noodles made from such starchy raw materials as wheat, mung beans, pea-starch and buckwheat, the latter sometimes blended with green tea, a rich source of catechins that act as antioxidants and free radical scavengers (see p. 94).

Dairy products, including whole-fat cow's milk, cream, cheese and butter, all of which are high in saturated fat, play almost no role in Japanese cookery. Meat is almost a condiment. It is shredded or cut into tiny pieces to flavour a dish of noodles or rice and is eaten in smaller quantities than in the West.

For protein, Japanese cooks often rely on the highly nutritious soya bean. In a process similar to cheese making, the beans are boiled down into a milk and the curds, known as tofu, are then formed into small blocks. Other vegetables are eaten raw or cooked only lightly by stir-frying, which preserves valuable nutrients.

Provisions from the sea

For most Japanese, a major source of nourishment is the sea that surrounds their islands. Virtually every sea creature obtainable finds its way onto the Japanese table: squid and octopus, shellfish of all descriptions, oily-fleshed fish such as mackerel, bonito, tuna and conger eel. As long as the fish is fresh and comes from pure, unpolluted water, Japanese delicacies of raw fish have all the virtues to delight a nutritionist's heart: they are high in protein, vitamins and valuable minerals such as calcium and zinc, rich in omega-3 polyunsaturated fats and low in saturated fats. The sea is also a

A gift of health from the sea

Coastal dwellers worldwide have always prized seaweed as a rich source of nutrients. These 'sea vegetables' come in many varieties, from crinkly purplish dulse to deep green sheets of nori and dark strands of hiziki. Although high in sodium, they boast a wealth of amino acids, vitamin B_{12} (one of the few sources in the plant world) and minerals including calcium, potassium and iodine.

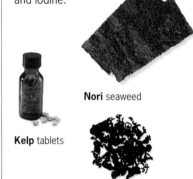

Nori seaweed

Kelp tablets

Fueru wakami

A TASTE OF THE OCEAN
The marine flavour of seaweed adds an intriguing note to rice dishes and stir-fries. It is available, dried, in health food shops or – for the less adventurous – can be purchased in tablet form

---

COOKING WITH TOFU

A delicate, silky substance, tofu is one of the most versatile materials in the Japanese larder: it can be steeped in an aromatic marinade and then grilled, stir-fried or simmered with other ingredients in broths. With only the subtlest flavour of its own, tofu readily takes on the taste of a sauce or any other ingredients that accompany it.

In addition to protein, tofu provides iron, calcium and B vitamins. It contains little saturated fat and no cholesterol.

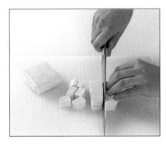

1 Using a sharp knife, slice the block of tofu into several strips. Then, keeping the strips together, slice them into 1.5 cm (½ in) cubes.

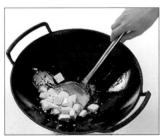

2 Heat a little oil in a wok. Add some chopped garlic and cook for 30 seconds. Add the tofu in batches, stir until lightly browned, then remove.

3 Add vegetables and sauces. Cook for 2 minutes. Stir in the tofu and stir-fry gently for 2 minutes. Serve with noodles.

Tofu, lightly stir-fried with mangetout, spring onions, carrots, sweet peppers and mushrooms, and sprinkled with sesame seeds, makes a delicious, healthy meal

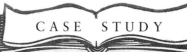
The Meat and Potatoes Man

People who have always eaten an American or northern European-style diet, with large portions of meat, high-fat dairy products and limited use of fresh vegetables and grains, often find it difficult to adopt a lighter, healthier diet. Learning to cook in Mediterranean style, however, offers many health benefits without too much effort.

Bill, aged 44, lives alone in a city-centre flat. Most of his dinners consist of a large helping of red meat, potatoes with butter and canned carrots. His usual lunch is a tuna and mayonnaise sandwich. When he works a late shift, he prepares a supper of eggs fried in butter, several rashers of bacon and thickly buttered toast. His father, who is in his early sixties, has recently suffered a stroke and has been told by his doctor that a lifelong diet high in saturated fats may have been a contributing factor. Bill has read articles about the positive benefits of Mediterranean meals, and now wants to try cooking them himself.

WHAT SHOULD BILL DO?

Bill should drastically cut down on his use of butter. He can still have a little on his toast, but should start using vegetable oils for sautés or salad dressings. Bill also must eat much smaller quantities of meat, using it in combination with pulses and fresh vegetables. He should look around his supermarket for types of fish that need little preparation, for example, salmon steaks, or mackerel fillets. Finally, Bill needs to increase his culinary repertoire. Newspapers and magazines often feature easy-to-prepare dishes, and there are plenty of cookbooks that contain Mediterranean recipes.

Action Plan

HEALTH
Visit a doctor to check blood cholesterol levels. Avoid full-fat dairy products, which are high in saturated fat.

DIET
Buy vegetables that can be eaten raw in salads, such as tomatoes and carrots, or can be cooked quickly, such as green beans.

EATING HABITS
Experiment with various foods that can be cooked quickly, such as foil-wrapped trout.

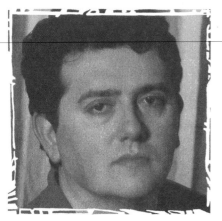

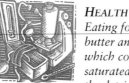

HEALTH
Eating foods such as butter and beef, which contain saturated fats, has the detrimental effect of raising blood cholesterol levels.

DIET
Canned vegetables and fruits should only be used when fresh or frozen are not readily available. With the exception of canned beans and peas, a high percentage of vitamins is lost in the canning process.

EATING HABITS
Although frying foods may be quick it is a very high-fat cooking method.

HOW THINGS TURNED OUT FOR BILL

Although Bill's cholesterol levels were not dangerously high, his doctor told him to reduce his intake of saturated fats. Bill's supermarket stocks some fresh vegetables, such as spinach, that are ready to cook, which Bill now buys instead of canned varieties. Bill has also found a lighter, Mediterranean way of cooking eggs. One egg, mixed with onions, peppers and diced cooked ham makes the Italian omelette known as frittata. But he does occasionally have eggs and bacon when the pressure at work has been high.

source of 'vegetables' for the Japanese, who delight in the numerous varieties of seaweed that grow around their coastlines and use their salty, marine intensity to season many of their dishes.

Flavours of the East

Many of the virtues of the Japanese diet are also found in the culinary traditions of China, Japan's neighbour across the Yellow Sea. It is impossible to speak of a single Chinese cuisine: each region of this enormous and populous landmass has its own distinctive cuisine, its own preferred ingredients and characteristic tastes. The intense, spicy-hot flavours of the western region of Szechuan, for instance, stand in marked contrast to the delicately flavoured and subtly blended seafood and vegetable combinations enjoyed by the Cantonese of the southeast. But there are common characteristics. Like the Japanese, the Chinese derive the bulk of their nourishment from carbohydrates – grains such as rice and millet, and wheat made into noodles or into a variety of steamed breads or buns.

Some of the features that make a Chinese diet healthy are the result of thousands of years of scarcity and the need to conserve

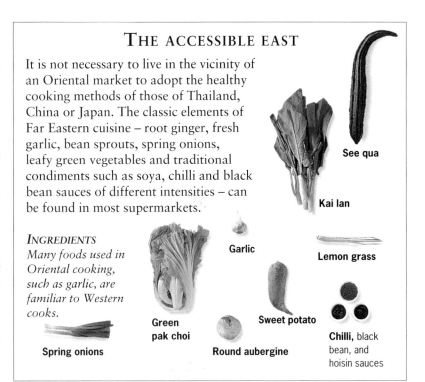

THE ACCESSIBLE EAST

It is not necessary to live in the vicinity of an Oriental market to adopt the healthy cooking methods of those of Thailand, China or Japan. The classic elements of Far Eastern cuisine – root ginger, fresh garlic, bean sprouts, spring onions, leafy green vegetables and traditional condiments such as soya, chilli and black bean sauces of different intensities – can be found in most supermarkets.

INGREDIENTS
Many foods used in Oriental cooking, such as garlic, are familiar to Western cooks.

See qua

Kai lan

Garlic

Lemon grass

Sweet potato

Green pak choi

Round aubergine

Chilli, black bean, and hoisin sauces

Spring onions

precious resources. The classic Chinese technique of stir-frying – the use of a small amount of oil, heated in a round-bottomed vessel called a wok, for high-speed cooking of thinly sliced or diced ingredients – is a good example. This method emerged, in part, from a need to conserve fuel in a land that had little wood, or other combustible energy sources to burn. But the benefits go beyond economy and ecology: the vegetable oils used in stir-frying are mainly polyunsaturated, and the cooking itself so swift that few nutrients are lost.

Steaming is another energy-efficient and healthful Chinese cooking method. Flat-bottomed, openweave bamboo baskets are stacked on top of one another and placed over a vessel filled with boiling water. As the steam rises, it cooks the foods on each tier as it passes through; since no liquid touches the food, very few nutrients leach into the water.

One common element of these diets is their ingenious use of a few simple ingredients. Combining small amounts of meat or fish with lightly cooked vegetables and plentiful amounts of rice or noodles, and adding distinctive herbs and spices, makes a little protein go a long way. The results bring together the delights and virtues of the Far Eastern diet: fresh flavours, health-giving ingredients and very little fat.

EATING FISH RAW

For Japanese cooks, the freshness of fish is paramount. No fishmonger in the world has to face a fussier set of customers, especially when the seafood is destined to be served in the celebrated assemblages of raw fish known as sushi and sashimi.

EXOTIC TASTES
Sushi is a carefully crafted parcel of bits of fresh fish pressed into lightly vinegared rice flavoured with soy sauce. Sashimi is an array of thinly sliced seafood.

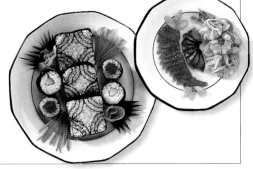

EQUIPMENT
Oriental cooking techniques require some pieces of equipment that differ from those used by Western cooks. But utensils such as woks and steamers are available in most cookware shops.

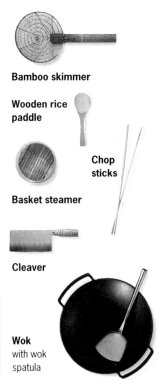

Bamboo skimmer

Wooden rice paddle

Chop sticks

Basket steamer

Cleaver

Wok
with wok spatula

MEETING YOUR FAMILY'S NEEDS

Different amounts of specific nutrients are required at each stage of life. And, as people grow and mature, lifestyles change, with the result that everyone has a unique set of nutritional needs.

An energetic toddler, an adolescent experiencing growth spurts, a pregnant woman, an adult who spends several hours a day sitting at a desk, another adult who earns a living out of doors in a physically demanding trade, a parent who goes out to work and returns home to the second full-time job of running a house and a family, a woman going through the menopause, an elderly person – all these people differ in the amounts and types of energy they expend and in the kinds of nutrients they require to keep themselves healthy.

Active, healthy infants and small children need a high number of calories in their small intake of food. Consequently, infants and young children can eat a larger amount of calorie-rich fats than middle-aged adults. Because fats deliver, gram for gram, virtually twice as much energy as proteins or carbohydrates, they are a valuable source of calories for a young body, which requires an enormous amount of energy to grow and thrive. Five to six-year-old children need at least 1710 calories a day. Most nutritionists also believe that children, like adults, should avoid an excessive consumption of saturated fats in favour of monounsaturated or polyunsaturated fats.

A LIFETIME OF DIFFERENCES

During infancy and early childhood, the body grows and develops at a phenomenal rate; virtually every intellectual and physical

MEALS FOR A TODDLER

Although a toddler's food intake is small and may be limited to a few foodstuffs, he or she requires, per body size, more fat and nutrients than the rest of the family.

Wholewheat cereal with full-fat milk provides fibre and calcium

Minced lean meat is a rich source of iron

Mashed potato with cheese provides carbohydrate, protein and fat

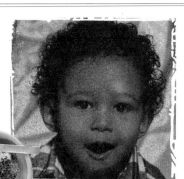

Bananas supply fibre; cottage cheese is protein-rich

Eggs are a valuable source of quality protein but must always be well cooked. Serve on a bed of salad, which provides vitamin C

FUSSY EATERS
Toddlers can be very picky eaters. Make foods more appealing by presenting them in interesting shapes and colours.

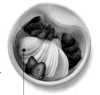

Pear and strawberries offer fibre and vitamin C

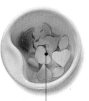

Cheddar cheese is a concentrated source of protein, fat and calcium

Yoghurt and fruit milkshake supplies protein, fat, calcium and vitamins

Pasta and vegetable soup is a good source of complex carbohydrates

faculty is being stretched and exercised. And, as anyone who has ever been surrounded by a roomful of preschool-age children knows, toddlers are capable of sustaining a fierce and furious level of physical activity, never walking when they can run, rarely speaking when they can shout, and moving frantically from one new source of stimulation to another.

The middle-aged male, however, no matter how active his lifestyle, no longer needs a hefty intake of calories for growth. If he does find himself growing at all, it is, inevitably, an unwelcome expansion around his waistline. And, apart from the relatively small percentage of the population working in highly demanding physical jobs, for example as a labourer on a building site or a farm hand, many middle-aged men are engaged in occupations requiring little expenditure of physical energy. They sit while they travel to work – in a car or on a train or a bus – and are likely to remain seated throughout much of the working day and possibly for most of their leisure hours.

For this reason, the calorie intake that turns the child into a powerhouse of healthy growth becomes, in a middle-aged man or postmenopausal woman, a dangerous cargo of excess nutritional baggage. It increases their risk of heart disease, hypertension and stroke and imposes an unhealthy burden on the circulatory system. Conscientious efforts to eat a balanced diet and exercise regularly are essential for keeping fit and healthy. But they will never be able to assimilate the equivalent amount of calories, taken as a percentage of body size, that are taken in and burned up daily by a lively, healthy five-year-old child.

A vital role

Faced with the different nutritional needs of every member of the family, health-conscious cooks may well feel as if they have been thrust under the spotlight in a circus ring to perform a juggling act involving several different meals, consisting of different ingredients and served at different times. But the task is not as daunting as it seems at first glance. The essential thing is to remember that everyone, whatever age, gender or lifestyle, will benefit from a balanced, varied diet that is well supplied with complex carbohydrates, especially whole grains and fresh vegetables and fruit. These foods are

MEALS FOR A TEENAGER

Many adolescents eat a high-fat diet, which provides them with plenty of energy. But, like everybody else, it is important that they have a good intake of fresh fruits and vegetables.

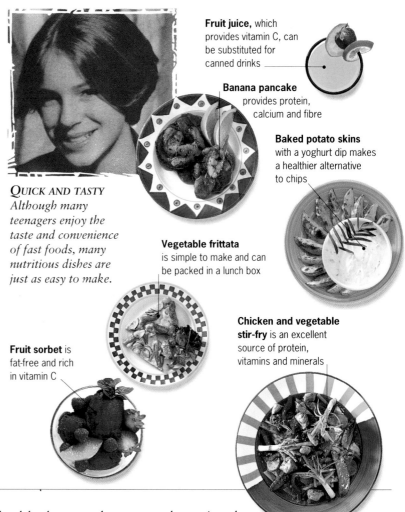

QUICK AND TASTY
Although many teenagers enjoy the taste and convenience of fast foods, many nutritious dishes are just as easy to make.

Fruit juice, which provides vitamin C, can be substituted for canned drinks

Banana pancake provides protein, calcium and fibre

Baked potato skins with a yoghurt dip makes a healthier alternative to chips

Vegetable frittata is simple to make and can be packed in a lunch box

Fruit sorbet is fat-free and rich in vitamin C

Chicken and vegetable stir-fry is an excellent source of protein, vitamins and minerals

healthy because they are moderate in salt and sugar content, low in saturated fats and good sources of vitamins and minerals.

Some members of the family (for example, a diabetic) may need special foods to fill particular nutritional needs; others will do better simply to skip particular foods, or cut down and eat a little less than habit dictates. But no matter what the variations in personal requirements or preferences, it is not necessary to transform your kitchen into a full-service restaurant, providing completely different menus for each person in the household. Simply knowing the people you live with and taking a few minutes to consider their different needs, are the most important steps you can take.

continued on page 124

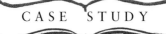
A Multi-Generational Family

The task of providing healthy meals for a family that may span three generations is a considerable challenge, particularly since the individual members of that family will have special lifestyles, particular health concerns and varying likes and dislikes. In many families, the person responsible for feeding the family may well be juggling this task with the demands of a full-time or part-time job.

Anne Martin, who is 38 years old, and her husband, Peter, who is 46, have three children: baby Jess, who has just celebrated her first birthday, eight-year-old David, and Erica, aged 14. The family also includes Anne's 72-year-old father, Tom, who has been living with the Martin family for three years, since the death of Anne's mother.

Peter commutes by train to his job as office manager for an insurance company. Anne works part-time as an admissions clerk at the local hospital, so Jess spends Monday to Friday mornings at a daycare centre.

The two older children have a busy after-school schedule. David is a Cub Scout, and Erica has become the star sprinter for the girls' athletics team at her school. Anne worries that Peter, who spends so much of his day sitting down, is not getting enough exercise. The results of his sedentary lifestyle, coupled with the high-fat lunches in the office canteen, are beginning to show around his waistline. Working in a hospital, she has seen men even younger than her husband suffering from heart problems and heart attacks. She also is concerned about her father, who,

although he seems in reasonably good health for his age, suffers from constipation. And Anne worries about her children's nutrition. She was alarmed to discover, when she took the baby for her last checkup, that Jess is slightly underweight for her age. Anne also knows that a lively eight-year-old and a teenage athlete need a well-balanced diet that will give them plenty of energy. Steering them away from junk food sometimes seems like a losing battle, especially with a young son who regards most fresh vegetables as a hostile alien life form.

CHILDREN
A study at the Children's Nutrition Center of the University of Texas found that 9 to 11-year-olds who missed breakfast performed less well on problem-solving exercises than those who ate an early morning meal.

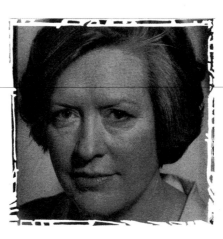

TEENAGERS
The enormous appetites of adolescents often go hand in hand with a social life that centres on the consumption of food notoriously high in fat or sugar: fast-food burgers, chips, ice cream and soft drinks.

FAMILY MEALS
A high-fat diet, coupled with an inactive lifestyle, may lead to serious health problems in adults, such as heart disease. But children often need the extra calories provided by fat.

TIME PRESSURES
Cooking with cereals, grains and fresh vegetables is more labour-intensive than simply slipping a couple of steaks or chops under the grill or into the frying pan.

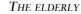

THE ELDERLY
Older people may suffer from a lack of iron, calcium and certain vitamins. It is believed, for instance, that one of the side effects of ageing is a decrease in the body's ability to retain vitamin C.

WHAT SHOULD ANNE DO?

Anne should begin by accepting that she is not the only person responsible for the entire family's well-being: every member of the household, apart from tiny Jess, is capable of understanding the importance of eating healthily and thinking about ways to improve his or her own diet. Rather than imposing rules that they will ignore, Anne should call a family conference to discuss the situation.

Instead of feeling guilty, Anne should start by thinking positively about the things she does right. For instance, she knows the importance of a good breakfast and makes the ingredients available to her family. She recognises the need to cut down on the consumption of animal fats and simple carbohydrates, is aware of everyone's need for plenty of foods high in fibre and appreciates the benefits of eating more fresh vegetables and fruit.

When the whole family are together, Anne should get them to suggest new, healthy recipes that they can try out over the next few weeks. She should also establish a rota so that each person helps her to work out the shopping lists for the week.

To arouse the children's interest in food, Anne should ask the most artistic junior member of the household to decorate a scrapbook, large folder or box-file, for storing healthy eating ideas and recipes found in newspapers and magazines.

Action Plan

CHILDREN
For breakfast, offer wholegrain, high-fibre cereals instead of sugary flakes with lower nutritional value. Serve fruit or fruit juice at breakfast. Muesli bars could be substituted for biscuits. Ask David what he would like to eat for lunch.

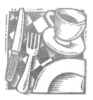

TEENAGERS
Stock up on the basics for healthy snacks: crunchy vegetables for eating raw, such as carrot and celery sticks, cucumbers and cherry tomatoes; low or reduced-fat dairy products, such as yoghurt and low-fat cottage cheese; and healthy nibbles, such as raisins and unsalted nuts.

FAMILY MEALS
Encourage Peter to give up his canteen lunches and take a low-fat lunch to work at least four times a week. Cut down on the use of meat as a main ingredient and, apart from Jess, drink only low-fat milk. Offer Jess more full-fat dairy products, such as yoghurt flavoured with fresh fruit.

TIME PRESSURES
Experiment with two timesaving 'cook-in-advance' sessions every week, to prepare large batches of vegetable soups, and vegetable-rich stews – such as red-bean chilli. Such ready-to-eat meals will give the family a healthy and appealing alternative to fast-food meals.

THE ELDERLY
Make cooked fruit dishes and buy bananas, berries and peaches for grandfather Tom, who has false teeth and finds chewing crunchy fruits, such as apples, difficult. Encourage Tom to visit the dentist to sort out his denture problems. Urge him to eat wholemeal breads and rolls.

HOW THINGS TURNED OUT FOR ANNE

A few months into this new regime, Anne feels she has the situation somewhat more under control. The baby is gaining more weight, and her husband, to Anne's great relief, is not, although she wishes he would take exercise regularly. The switch to wholemeal breads has had an unexpected spin-off: Anne's father, convinced that no one makes bread the way he remembers it from his boyhood, has developed an interest in baking various breads himself and now spends happy hours providing the family's weekly bread supply. Anne wonders secretly if his improved temperament also has something to do with the digestive improvements caused by more fibre in his diet. The family's resolve to try as many new vegetable dishes and salads as possible has turned up a number of things that even her son with his hatred of vegetables will eat, but Anne still finds herself fighting a losing battle in her efforts to ensure that David eats a healthy lunch. At school, he tends to swap his apple and sandwiches for someone else's chocolate biscuit and chips. And no matter how many healthy treats are in the refrigerator, the two older children are as likely as ever to glance at them and complain that there is nothing in there to eat.

MEALS FOR A PREGNANT WOMAN

When expecting a baby, a woman needs extra protein and almost twice as much calcium as usual.

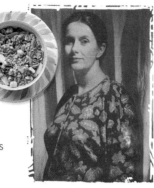

Cheese and ham omelette is high in protein and calcium

Muesli with semi-skimmed milk offers fibre and calcium

Fresh fruit salad supplies vitamin C; yoghurt has plenty of calcium

DEVELOPING FOETUS
A good intake of calcium is vital while the baby's teeth and skeletal system are being formed. Protein is needed for the laying down of new tissue.

Chicken wrapped in cabbage with couscous is a good source of protein, vitamin C and carbohydrate

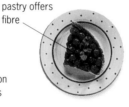

Raspberry tart supplies vitamin C and the wholemeal pastry offers fibre

Greens provide folic acid, which helps to prevent birth defects

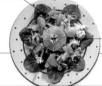

Oranges are full of vitamin C, which aids the absorption of iron from carbohydrates and pulses

The growing body

The basic principles of a healthy diet remain the same throughout life, but children, especially from infancy to the age of seven, have particular nutritional needs to support their development and promote good health. For example, even though whole milk is higher in saturated fats, nutritionists believe that babies and young children should drink it instead of skimmed milk to ensure they are not missing out on vital nutrients. The goal is to wean children onto semi-skimmed milk, then skimmed milk by the age of seven.

Protein, too, because of its vital role in growth, is particularly important for the young. Adults and older children naturally produce all but eight of the amino acids that make up protein; they must obtain these missing elements from food. Babies and small children, however, lack another one or two of the essential amino acids, so they need to consume more high-quality protein, such as dairy products and poultry, to make up the shortfall. According to nutritionists, children between one and three years require 0.81 grams of protein per pound of their own body weight every day, while those between seven and ten years need only 0.55 grams. Adults, in contrast, require only 0.36 grams, less than half the amount recommended for the very young.

A pregnant woman or one who is breast-feeding a baby also has special needs, since what she eats has an effect on her child's

SPORTING REQUIREMENTS

Athletes who make frequent and often punishing demands on their physical resources have special dietary needs beyond those of the ordinary person who exercises for good health.

For a long time it was believed that a large intake of protein was essential for athletic success – would-be Olympic champions and boxing contenders would fuel their training efforts with huge steaks for breakfast. While protein is important – especially for the repair of damaged tissue, such as the strains acquired on the sports field – current nutritional thinking emphasises the intake of unrefined complex carbohydrates as a source of energy. The aspiring track star

is now more likely to eat huge helpings of wholemeal pasta to stoke up with fuel for a forthcoming marathon.

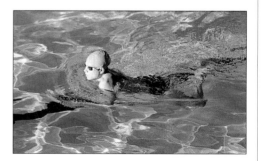

SUSTAINING ENERGY
To ensure a steady supply of energy during competition, athletes eat a variety of complex carbohydrate foods before the event.

development. To help sustain the baby's growth and her own good health, she needs an iron-rich diet, with foods that are plentiful in vitamin B_6 and folic acid – for example, spinach, cauliflower, broccoli, brussels sprouts, cabbage and beans. And because the formation of the baby's bones and teeth will leach away her own supply of calcium, she needs to keep up her intake by drinking sufficient reduced-fat milk and eating calcium-rich foods such as yoghurt or sardines (with the bones).

The ravenous age

Teenagers' needs also differ from those of their elders. The constantly ravenous adolescent, trawling the refrigerator, is a familiar sight in many families. If based on healthy foods, the frequent snacks between meals that teenagers crave will help to supply the complex nutritional needs of a growing body passing through puberty. But the greatest challenge for the parents of a healthy adolescent is to ensure that the snack foods their son or daughter chooses will actually do some good. Processed products and greasy fast foods, which are high in saturated fat, salt and sugar, are easy options for the teenager in a hurry and may lead to poor nutritional habits that will be difficult to break and result in health problems, such as heart disease, in middle age.

For the teenager's parents, the consumption of frequent snacks could be a sure step on the road to obesity. Men of average height and frame need only approximately 2750 calories a day, while women, because of a generally smaller build, are advised to consume a slightly lower intake – approximately 2150 calories daily.

Slowing down

Nutritional requirements change sooner than one might think – at about the age of 35. Metabolism slows down, and people often become less physically active, so calorie intake should be scaled down accordingly, or exercise increased. A sedentary man in his sixties needs approximately 2330 calories a day, while a woman in her sixties needs about 1900 calories.

By a conscious adjustment of their dietary habits, such as cutting down their intake of foods high in fat, cholesterol, salt and refined carbohydrates, and by eating plenty of foods high in fibre, adults can protect themselves not only against becoming overweight but also against many of the illnesses that accompany ageing. Current nutritional thinking, for example, suggests that all adults should consume an average of 18 grams of dietary fibre daily, in the form of fresh fruits, vegetables and wholegrain cereals or wholemeal breads; an elderly person might choose to increase this total to help combat constipation.

RESTRICTED DIETS

Whatever the age of family members, their individual circumstances may also vary. Vegetarians who do not eat meat or poultry but may possibly eat fish, and vegans, who eat no animal products of any kind, including dairy products, have special nutritional needs, since they have to obtain most or all of their protein, calcium and B vitamins from non-animal sources.

A family member who is trying to lose weight by following a calorie-controlled diet, depends not only on self-discipline, but also on the cooperation of anyone involved

MEALS FOR A MIDDLE-AGED PERSON

The risk of heart disease increases dramatically once an adult reaches middle age.

Pure fruit spread contains natural sugars

Mackerel offers important fatty acids that help to prevent heart disease

Potatoes are a valuable source of carbohydrate

Beetroot provides carotenoids, which are antioxidants

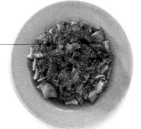

HEALTHY HEART
To reduce the risk of heart disease, a diet low in saturated fats is vital. Also eat foods rich in antioxidants (see p. 94).

Ratatouille is made with monounsaturated olive oil

Fresh fruit salad has a good supply of the antioxidant vitamin C

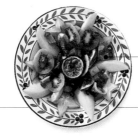

MEALS FOR AN ELDERLY PERSON

As a person grows older, extra fibre may be needed to prevent constipation. Some older people experience a diminished sense of taste and should guard against an overuse of salt.

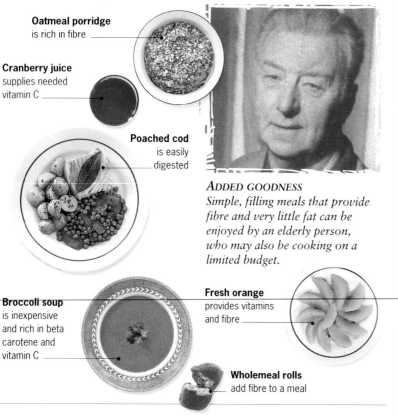

Oatmeal porridge
is rich in fibre

Cranberry juice
supplies needed
vitamin C

Poached cod
is easily
digested

ADDED GOODNESS
Simple, filling meals that provide fibre and very little fat can be enjoyed by an elderly person, who may also be cooking on a limited budget.

Broccoli soup
is inexpensive
and rich in beta
carotene and
vitamin C

Fresh orange
provides vitamins
and fibre

Wholemeal rolls
add fibre to a meal

in cooking and shopping to ensure that meals contain the right balance of the foods they need and to keep unhealthy, fattening temptations to a minimum.

Others may have dietary restrictions based on illness or high cholesterol. Certain medical conditions, such as diabetes or hypertension, require special consideration in planning and cooking meals and in the actual shopping for ingredients. Scrupulous label reading is necessary, for instance, to ensure that a person suffering from hypertension – whose well-being may depend on a reduction of salt in the diet – is not being bombarded with the 'hidden' salts found in so many processed and packaged foods. And a diabetic may not only need to restrict the intake of particular foods, such as sugar, but may have to pay special attention to the timing and composition of meals. Someone convalescing after serious illness, who may have a weakened immune system, also needs to receive the nutrients, such as proteins, vitamins and minerals, that boost recovery and promote good health.

BURNING CALORIES

Even for people with no specific health concerns, differences in lifestyle have definite implications for diet. The caloric needs of a labourer doing heavy manual work far outstrip those of the deskbound. Since dietary

A SNACK AT HAND

HEALTHY INDULGENCE
Keep on hand a good supply of fruit and vegetables, nuts, seeds and wholewheat products to satisfy between-meal cravings.

The key to satisfying the needs and tastes of all family members can be found not only on the dinner table but also in the refrigerator and the store cupboard.

The foods snack-hungry youngsters eat between meals are as important as those they consume around the family dinner table. Be sure always to have on hand a bowl laden with the most colourful array

of fruit that the season can provide; a selection of unsweetened wholegrain cereals, ready to eat with a little low-fat milk; a container, kept in the refrigerator, full of ready-to-eat raw vegetables, such as carrot sticks, cucumber sticks and crisp wedges of red, green and yellow peppers; and a supply of medium-fat or low-fat cheeses, such as cottage cheese or feta.

**Paw paw and
kiwifruits** are good
sources of vitamin C

**Dried
bananas**
contain the
mineral potassium

Pistachio nuts
are high in protein

Sunflower seeds
provide vitamin E

Carrots, tomatoes and red
and green peppers are rich in
the antioxidants vitamin C
and beta carotene

**Low-fat cottage
cheese** is a source
of protein

**Wholewheat
biscuits** supply
fibre

**Feta cheese and
salad in pitta bread**
make a nourishing
high-fibre, low-fat snack

fat contains twice the calories as the same weight of protein, only adults who burn up an enormous number of calories are likely to be able to sustain a high-fat diet without becoming overweight. For the average individual, nutritionists recommend that fat should provide no more than 30 per cent of calorie intake, with a maximum of 10 per cent of this fat consumption coming from saturated fats.

Nevertheless, anyone who has worked in a sedentary job, with set hours and a comparatively unchanging routine, knows how difficult it is to avoid the temptation to break up the routine of the working day with a quick foray to the nearest source of potato crisps, chocolate bars and soft drinks. But whenever you do succumb, you should adjust your daily calorie intake accordingly, since a can of cola or a chocolate bar can provide more than the maximum recommended simple carbohydrate intake for an entire day. Alternatively, keep some healthy foods, such as dried fruits and wholemeal biscuits, in your bag or office drawer to help satisfy the urge for a snack.

PACKING HEALTH INTO A LUNCH BOX

The following tips can help you to provide the members of your family with nourishing, tasty foods during their lunch breaks.

▶ *For sandwich fillings, use skinless chicken or turkey breast meat, instead of fatty luncheon meats or sausages such as salami. Moisten wholemeal bread with a smear of ketchup or mild mustard instead of butter or mayonnaise, and add crunch by lining the bread with crisp lettuce leaves and green peppers.*

▶ *Reduce the fat in a tuna salad sandwich by using tuna packed in brine and replacing half the mayonnaise with low-fat yoghurt.*

▶ *For a nutritious, vegetarian sandwich spread, mix a small amount of peanut butter with a mashed banana.*

FEEDING A FAMILY

The best strategy for feeding a group of people with different needs is to plan meals around the common denominators, and then add extras for those who need additional nutrients. A typical basic menu, for instance, might consist of wholemeal pasta with a sauce made of onions, tomatoes, peppers, mushrooms and fresh herbs, accompanied by a leafy green salad, with a platter of fresh fruits and low-fat yoghurt for dessert.

For someone who requires more protein – or is a determined meat eater – make the salad more substantial by adding some lean cooked chicken or turkey. Fish, especially tuna or sardines, would add cholesterol-busting omega-3 acids as well.

A generous handful of bean sprouts, alfalfa sprouts, mung beans or chickpeas or a sprinkling of sesame seeds or wheatgerm will also boost protein.

Drinking a glass of milk with the meal will provide extra calcium for those who need it, for example, a pregnant woman or very young child. And both the pasta and the salad can be accompanied by small dishes of supplementary garnishes, to be added as needed.

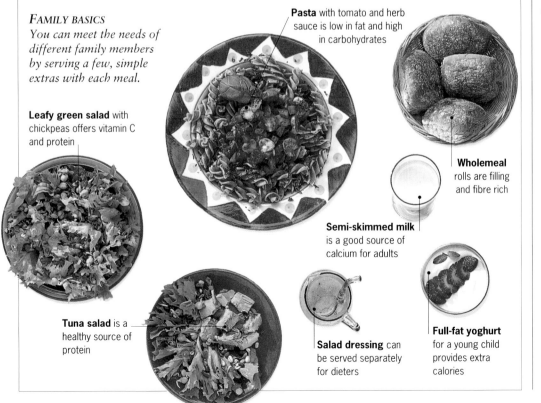

FAMILY BASICS
You can meet the needs of different family members by serving a few, simple extras with each meal.

Leafy green salad with chickpeas offers vitamin C and protein

Pasta with tomato and herb sauce is low in fat and high in carbohydrates

Wholemeal rolls are filling and fibre rich

Semi-skimmed milk is a good source of calcium for adults

Tuna salad is a healthy source of protein

Salad dressing can be served separately for dieters

Full-fat yoghurt for a young child provides extra calories

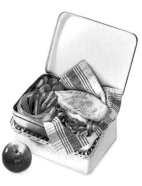

READY TO EAT
Tuck in some easy-to-eat raw vegetables, fresh fruit, dried fruits such as apricots, and sandwiches made with wholemeal pitta bread.

COOKING FOR YOUR CHILDREN

Children grow so fast that they need a higher proportion of nutrients in their diets than adults. They often prefer refined foods, however, and can sometimes be very picky eaters.

Children may refuse to eat for many reasons, few of which have to do with the food. Although your children may reject certain foods, if you offer a variety of nutritious foods that are cooked or presented in an appealing manner, you will find things they like that are good for them. If you are unsure about the nutritional content of your children's diet, contact your doctor for advice.

Problems with eating hot food

The flavour and texture of many foods will change when they are cooked and some children will baulk at the difference. This change most often happens with vegetables. Children may gobble up raw carrots, for example, but ignore them cooked. If this is the case with your children, let them eat cleaned raw vegetables. They generally have a higher vitamin and mineral content than cooked vegetables and are a good source of fibre. Introduce other cooked foods until you find some that your child likes.

Be patient and bear in mind that if your child is thriving – has an abundance of energy, sleeps well, is not underweight or overweight and does not suffer from stomach cramps, constipation or diarrhoea – then he or she is developing well.

HEIGHT AND WEIGHT CHARTS FOR CHILDREN

Growth charts help you to check whether your child is developing healthily. The solid green and purple 'percentile' lines identify average height or weight at a given age, the dotted red and orange lines indicate the high and low ends of the normal range. Ninety-six per cent of all children's height or weight falls within the dotted lines. To monitor your child's development, request a chart from your paediatrician.

GROWTH CURVES
Your child's measurements, when plotted regularly, should form a natural curve roughly parallel to the average (50th percentile). Children generally progress in line with their height and weight at birth. For example, if your child's height is above average at birth, then his or her weight curve will also fall above the central one. There should be cause for concern only if the growth pattern veers away from the average curve.

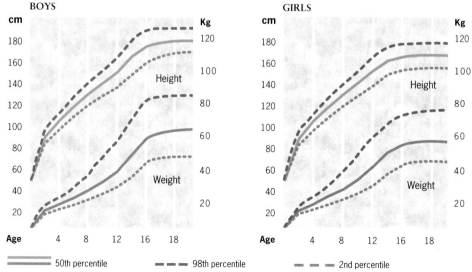

Improving the Household's Diet with a

Family Conference

The best way to rethink the family diet is by teamwork. Get everyone in the household involved by calling a conference. Turn the meeting into a special occasion that will be fun and enjoyed by all.

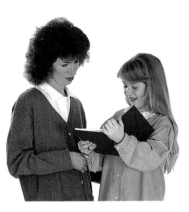

The place: the family kitchen or dining table. The time: a weekend hour or weekday evening when everyone can arrange to be free and at home. The refreshments: a medley of the family's favourite snacks.

The supplies: blank paper, felt-tip pens or pencils in different colours.
Appoint a note taker. Label different sheets of paper: Likes, Dislikes, Eat More, Eat Less, Special Needs, Healthy Snacks, Treats.

VALUABLE COMMUNICATION
Making time for a family discussion is a good way of looking at the healthy – and unhealthy – aspects of everyone's diet.

HOLDING THE CONFERENCE

Start talking! Discuss the way the family usually eats. Give everyone a chance to list his or her favourite foods, dishes and types of cooking, as well as the things he or she likes the least.

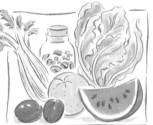

1 *Let everyone come up with suggestions for healthy foods that the family should eat more of, then a list of the items that should be cut down or eliminated altogether.*

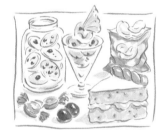

2 *Talk about the fun foods that everybody loves, but are too high in fats, sugars and certain additives to be truly healthy. Agree how often, and when, these special treats can be eaten.*

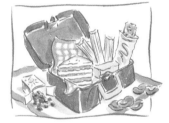

3 *Think about how to maintain the family's eating patterns away from home – the children's packed lunches or school meals, the adults' lunches at work or on business trips.*

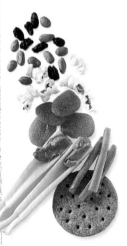

COMPETITION TIME
Ask for suggestions for healthy snacks to have on hand. Reward the family member who can contribute the greatest number of ideas.

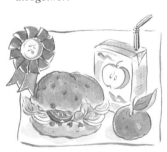

4 *Give a prize to the person who comes up with the best ideas for healthy eating in these situations – including suggestions by the family's junior members for foods to pack in their school lunch boxes that will not be traded or left uneaten.*

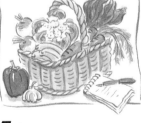

5 *Agree to try a new healthy recipe at regular intervals. Organise a menu-planning rota so that each person helps the household cook to think up the menus for a week's meals, work out the shopping lists and shop for the ingredients.*

BREAKFAST STRATEGY TIPS

▶ *Discuss the elements that make up a healthy breakfast; think about foods that are the easiest to put together when everyone is in a hurry.*

▶ *Simplify breakfast preparation in the morning by planning ahead – for example, set the table and put out dry cereals the night before.*

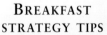

SPECIAL DIETS

A high proportion of the population follows some kind of special diet. Many people do so to lose weight, but a significant number follow a programme for medical reasons.

Special diets tend to fall into one of three broad categories. The first is the exclusion diet – particular foods are not eaten because of a food allergy or intolerance – for example, the gluten-free diet prescribed for people with coeliac disease, or the diet that excludes cow's milk products for lactose-intolerant individuals. The second category is the reduced-intake diet, in which less is eaten of certain elements that are likely to aggravate an existing health problem, such as a low-salt diet for people prone to hypertension. The third regime is an increased-consumption diet in which an individual eats more of foods that are believed to confer specific health benefits. For example, nutritional guidelines for post-menopausal women at risk of developing osteoporosis include an increased consumption of high-calcium foods, such as low-fat cheeses and milk, sardines and salmon (with the bones), pulses and leafy green vegetables.

GLUTEN-FREE DIET

One of the most common special diets is the gluten-free regime, prescribed for people who suffer from an extreme sensitivity to various grains. Gluten – a protein found in wheat, rye, barley and oats – is impossible for some people to absorb. A person's inability to absorb gluten, whether because of coeliac disease or any one of a number of related medical conditions, causes thickening and inflammation of the small bowel, which prevents absorption of nutrients. The problem is controlled by eliminating wheat, rye, barley and oats from the diet.

People with this sensitivity must cut out a wide range of foodstuffs, including all standard varieties of bread and pasta and most breakfast cereals. They must also become scrupulous and knowledgeable readers of food packaging and labels. Gluten in the form of 'wheat', 'flour', 'wheat starch' 'modified starch' and similar substances is a common additive in a wide variety of processed foods. It even turns up in canned soups and bottled sauces, although not every manufacturer uses it. Coeliac sufferers rapidly learn which brands to avoid, and organisations set up to support and advise people with this condition frequently publish lists of gluten-free products as well as recipes for bread substitutes and other dishes.

But even people with a high sensitivity to wheat need complex carbohydrates in their diets. Digestible carbohydrates in a gluten-free diet may come from grains such as rice or corn, which do not contain this particular protein. Health food shops and some supermarkets stock gluten-free breads, pastas and savoury biscuits, such as rice cakes, to take the place of the forbidden foods.

TREATING ARTHRITIS

Some medical practitioners, especially if they are involved in alternative or complementary medicine, believe that specific food sensitivities and allergies are responsible for a variety of ailments, and they often prescribe diets designed with these difficulties in mind.

Naturopaths, for example, recommend a high-alkaline diet to reduce the toxic acids that they believe accumulate in the joints of people suffering from arthritis. This regime, which is not included among the arthritis treatments normally advocated by orthodox medicine, bans some of the same substances, such as wheat flour and its derivatives, forbidden to people on gluten-free diets. It may also eliminate or severely curtail the intake of cow's milk, citrus fruits, salt, pepper and red meat. Some arthritics have found that avoiding all nightshade family foods – tomatoes, potatoes and aubergines – will often ease their symptoms within three weeks.

EASING INFLAMMATION Pineapples contain an enzyme called bromelain, which is thought to reduce inflammation caused by arthritis. Oily fish may also be helpful.

THE DIABETIC DIET

Diabetes is another medical condition that requires a carefully controlled diet. There are different kinds of diabetes, but their common denominator is a disruption of the body's ability to metabolise carbohydrates because of difficulties in the production of insulin, the hormone that controls the amount of sugar in the blood (see p. 48). A small percentage of diabetics need regular insulin injections, but most, especially those who have adult-onset diabetes, can stabilise their conditions through diet.

Diabetics are often advised to schedule their intake of food in accordance with the times of maximum insulin activity within the body, eating small meals of carefully controlled quantities at regular intervals throughout the day. They must also restrict their intake of added sugar; a common guideline is to limit their consumption to less than five per cent of their total daily caloric intake. To accommodate the needs of this relatively large section of the population, manufacturers now produce an extensive range of sugar-free products.

Obesity often goes hand in hand with diabetes, and for many diabetics a calorie-controlled weight-reduction diet and a regular exercise regime are fundamental to managing their condition. In general, the dietary recommendations for diabetics conform closely to the nutritional guidelines put forward by such organisations as the British Heart Foundation: a reduction of total fats in the diet to less than 30 per cent of all calories consumed, with saturated fats reduced to less than 10 per cent; a reduction in the intake of salt, high-cholesterol foods and alcohol; and a substantial increase in unrefined, complex carbohydrates, such as those found in whole grains and wholemeal breads, to about 55 per cent of total calories.

CUTTING DOWN ON SALT

Most special diets recommend a reduction in the intake of sodium, a component of salt and other ingredients.

Excessive salt in the diet is one of a number of factors believed to be associated with the development of hypertension. Obesity, high alcohol consumption, smoking, a stressful job or lifestyle and even heredity have also been implicated. Even though scientists have not yet been able to provide sufficient ironclad evidence that eating too much salt is a direct cause of hypertension, many studies have shown that a reduction in salt will help to decrease high blood pressure. Virtually everyone treated for hypertension is told to cut down on his or her intake of salt.

Washing added salt away
The added salt content of processed foods can be significantly reduced by rinsing them in running water. A study at Duke University, in North Carolina, USA, revealed that canned green beans, rinsed for one minute, lost 41 per cent of their sodium content. The same treatment removed 76 per cent of the salt added to canned tuna.

SODIUM CONTENT IN CONDIMENTS AND SEASONINGS

FOOD ITEM	AMOUNT	SODIUM (mg)
SEASONINGS		
Table salt	1 tsp	1965
Baking powder	1 tsp	472
Chilli powder	1 tsp	30
Garlic salt	1 tsp	1850
Horseradish	1 tbsp	182
Meat tenderiser	1 tsp	1750
Mustard	1 tsp	413
Green olives in brine	4	360
Onion salt	1 tsp	1620
SAUCES		
Chilli	1 tbsp	786
Ketchup	1 tbsp	489
Soy	1 tbsp	1716
Tabasco	1 tsp	131
Worcestershire	1 tbsp	360
SALAD DRESSINGS		
French	1 tbsp	282
Mayonnaise	1 tbsp	72
Thousand Island	1 tbsp	312

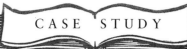
The Heart-Attack Survivor

Even a mild heart attack is a terrifying event for the victims and their families. It gives many survivors all the motivation they need to make fundamental and radical improvements in their diet and general lifestyle. Learning to eat healthily is essential for preventing further damage to the heart and for enjoying an active life.

George is a 45-year-old optician who runs his own practice. His wife, Charlotte, works with him. One morning, after a heavy snowfall, George began to shovel the snow off the pavement in front of his premises. But before he finished the task, he collapsed with severe chest pains and was taken to hospital where doctors diagnosed a heart attack. Fortunately, the attack was a relatively mild one, and George was told that after a period of rest and recovery, he should be able to resume work. However, his family doctor gave him a severe lecture about the need to change his eating habits, especially by cutting down on saturated fats. He put George on a low-fat diet, and warned him of the grave risks he would take if he failed to stick to it.

What should george do?

George and Charlotte should be sure to eat plenty of fresh vegetables and complex carbohydrates. If they want to grill something quickly during the week, they could choose fish, which is free of saturated fats. Their customary Sunday lunch has usually featured roast beef with roast potatoes. Since George and Charlotte have more time and energy for cooking on Sundays, this presents a good opportunity to experiment with some vegetarian recipes to substitute for the usual roast. Sandwiches for their weekday packed lunches should have fillings low in saturated fat, such as canned sardines mixed with a dash of lemon juice or vinegar. George should also avoid eating heavy meals within two hours of going to bed.

Action Plan

DIET
Give up beef (roast turkey is a much leaner, healthier substitute). Eat more oily fish, such as herrings. Use low-fat dairy products, such as reduced-fat mozzarella cheese.

COOKING METHODS
Try out some alternative cooking techniques, such as poaching skinless chicken or turkey. Boil or bake potatoes. Microwave, poach or steam fish rather than frying them.

FITNESS
Schedule regular, gentle exercise into the weekly routine. Possibilities include walking, swimming, gardening and yoga – choose one or more that he likes.

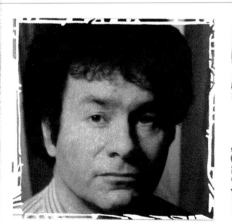

FITNESS
Self-employed people may have little leisure time for keeping fit and relaxing.

DIET
Red meats, even after trimming, contain considerable amounts of saturated fat. Some dairy products can also be harmful.

COOKING METHODS
Certain cooking techniques increase fat consumption. Frying is the method using the most fat, closely followed by roasting, if the meat is basted with the pan juices.

How things turned out for george

George has been back to the doctor for a checkup and he seems to be making a good recovery. Although fish and fresh salads now figure on the weekly menu, Charlotte still feels that she and her husband are eating too much meat. She tried replacing the Sunday roast with a vegetarian meal but he complained. She thinks this may be a losing battle. They have agreed, however, to one meatless meal per week.

The body only needs the amount of sodium found in about one gram of salt per day to function normally. Nutritional guidelines in many countries suggest that even people who are not at risk of hypertension should limit their daily consumption to a maximum of three grams (3000 milligrams or one and a half teaspoons) a day. People with high blood pressure should cut their intake even further.

A hidden ingredient

Sticking to a low-salt diet requires careful attention. Many people salt their food – some do this before they have tasted it – but salt also has a way of sneaking into our food. In the United States, for instance, researchers have established that salt added at the table accounts for only one-third of an individual's average consumption. The other two-thirds is eaten in processed foods. But salty snacks, such as potato crisps, are not the only culprits.

Salt has long been used as a preservative to keep food safe. Salted or smoked fish, pickled vegetables and cured meats – such as bacon and salami – have always contained salt to keep them from spoiling. In fact, government food standards specify quantities of salt for many foods, such as sausages. Manufacturers rely heavily – too heavily, most nutritionists would say – upon salt to enhance the flavour of foods. Canned vegetables and vegetable juices, canned or dried soups include salt and sodium, so always read the label carefully before you buy. Canned tuna packed in oil, for instance, has a lower salt content than the same fish packed in brine. Many manufacturers now supply low-salt or no-added-salt versions of their products.

In any purchase of packaged food, the low-salt shopper needs to read carefully the small print on the label. As well as noting the quantity of salt itself, watch out for sodium hiding in other ingredients: MSG (monosodium glutamate), brine, soya sauce, baking powder, hydrolysed vegetable protein, miso, bouillon, kelp and other seaweed products, sodium citrate, and such additives as the sweetener saccharin.

Learning to like less salt

The best strategy for cutting down on salt is to re-educate your taste buds to enjoy other natural flavours in food. By gradually reducing the amount of salt you add to food

SEASONING WITHOUT SALT

In the kitchen, make use of ingredients that provide flavour but no sodium. Draw upon garlic, onions, root ginger, vinegar, wine, fiery chilli peppers and the juice of lemons, oranges and other fruits. If you must use a prepared condiment, stick to lower-salt varieties or improvise salt-reduced substitutes: Worcestershire sauce, for instance, though hardly salt free, has much less sodium than most soya sauces, and packs an equally aromatic punch.

ENHANCING THE FLAVOUR
By choosing highly aromatic herbs and spices, you can add interest to meat dishes without noticing the loss of salt.

Dill, Bay leaves, Rosemary, Cumin seeds, Thyme, Mint, Star anise, Red wine, vinegar and lemon juice, Garlic cloves, Sage, Red and green chillies, Curry powder, Root ginger, Onion, Tarragon

over a period of days or weeks, you will become more sensitive to saltiness. After a few weeks of progressively decreasing the use of the salt shaker, an amount that would have once seemed just normal will make the food taste unpleasantly salty. Experiment with flavourful seasonings (see box above).

On a low-salt diet you face a challenge when eating in restaurant. Choose dishes that can be cooked to order, and ask the kitchen to prepare them without adding salt.

LOWERING CHOLESTEROL

If you are following a low-cholesterol diet, you have to be equally resolute. To cut down on the saturated fats that are the building blocks of the health-threatening type of cholesterol, you will have to banish certain foods altogether from everyday use. Full-fat dairy products, such as full-fat milk, are perilously high in saturated fats; they should be replaced by their low-fat or fat-free counterparts, such as skimmed milk. Replace butter with vegetable oils high in polyunsaturates, or olive oil, which is substantially monounsaturated (see p. 51).

Holding the salt

Cut down on sodium levels by limiting the amount of salt used in recipes. A recipe designed to serve four people should contain no more than a ¼ teaspoon of salt. This will add 0.13 grams (125 milligrams) of sodium to each helping, which is well within the recommended daily allowance.

133

USING FOOD TO LOSE WEIGHT

A weight-loss diet, in essence, is simply one in which the body takes in less energy in the form of calories than it expends. But there is nothing simple about the diet industry.

Hundreds and hundreds of magazine and newspaper articles, as well as a vast array of diet books, hold out the promise of delivering sure-fire methods for shedding fat and decreasing weight. Every city or town has its diet clubs and franchised vendors of purportedly foolproof weight-reduction schemes. Manufacturers of special diet foods, ranging from liquid high-protein substitute meals to appetite-killing confectionery bars and savoury snacks, make extravagant claims in order to sell hope to weight-conscious consumers. A few of these diets are based on sound nutritional advice. But many companies make exaggerated or overoptimistic claims.

People who follow recommendations to cut down on calories will lose weight, but it is easy to put the weight back on again if, out of boredom or hunger or for some other reason, you give up the diet.

THE LOW-CALORIE DIET
For generations of dieters, one of the most familiar regimes has been the low-calorie diet, which concentrates simply on cutting down the number of calories consumed on a day-to-day basis. Its adherents rarely let a mouthful pass their lips without first consulting a chart detailing the exact caloric intake for every single ingredient.

Calorie control is, indeed, important for anyone trying to lose weight, but the major failing of such a diet is its lack of emphasis on the need for a varied and balanced intake of foods to provide the full range of health-sustaining nutrients your body requires.

Low-calorie diets offer little to deter a rigid calorie counter with a sweet tooth, for instance, from abandoning a dinner altogether in favour of a large slab of thickly iced chocolate cake. This is justified on the premise that the individual has not exceeded the recommended maximum calories for the day. Nutritionists would not be surprised to discover that this extreme interpretation of calorie control failed to deliver the dieter's hoped-for weight loss nor to find the dieter complaining of low energy, irritability, constipation or vertigo.

FAT DISTRIBUTION IN MEN AND WOMEN

About 10 to 15 per cent of a man's weight consists of fat, while 20 to 25 per cent is average for most women. Fat is stored under the skin all over the body but it is most likely to accumulate on specific areas of the male and female bodies.

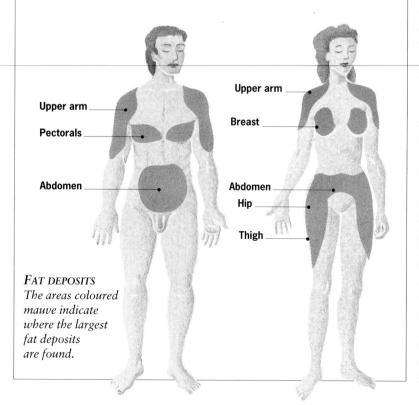

Upper arm

Pectorals

Abdomen

Upper arm

Breast

Abdomen

Hip

Thigh

FAT DEPOSITS
The areas coloured mauve indicate where the largest fat deposits are found.

BREAKING DOWN FAT

The places that fat settles in our bodies and the speed at which the body burns it up are controlled by hormones.

Oestrogen, the female sex hormone, mainly governs the deposits of fat around the hips and thighs; insulin – generated in the body via the consumption of carbohydrates – dictates the deposit of fat around the neck, shoulder blades and abdomen.

The body is an efficient ecosystem, however, and is constantly recycling its fat stores to provide the energy it needs.

Two stress hormones, adrenaline and noradrenaline, are responsible for releasing stored fat reserves when fresh energy is required. When these stress hormones go into operation, the fat deposits in certain parts of the body, such as the abdomen or the face, which are more sensitive to their presence, are recycled more readily and are the first to begin disappearing. For this reason, when weight loss does occur, the first visible signs for both males and females are likely to be a thinner face and a flatter stomach.

THE SPOT-REDUCTION DIET

A weight-loss programme that has become very fashionable and popular is the so-called spot-reduction diet. It promises the removal of unwanted excess fat from particular 'problem' areas, such as the hips or buttocks, through the combination of a low-fat diet and an exercise programme.

People who cut their consumption of fat and increase their amount of exercise will indeed have a good chance of losing weight, since fats – gram for gram – deliver a far heavier cargo of calories than the same quantity of protein or carbohydrate. But the notion that such a dieter can sculpt his or her body by a highly localised weight-reduction programme is wishful thinking.

Scientists at King's College, London, set up a study to compare the effectiveness of a spot-reduction diet to that of a standard weight-reduction diet that allowed a controlled daily intake of 1000 to 1200 calories. They asked two groups of women to follow each regime and then compared the results. Both groups lost poundage, but the weight loss followed the same pattern: most inches were lost from the waist rather than from the hips or thighs, as promised in the spot-reduction plan, and the women's busts became smaller as quickly as their hips did.

FOOD-COMBINING DIET

Another eating plan that is enjoying a surge of popularity is food-combining. This system operates by a strict set of rules governing the types of food that may – or may not – be eaten within the same meal. Weight loss is only a single aspect of the diet, which also claims to promote general good health.

By eating or avoiding certain foods at certain times, the dieter supposedly purges the body of harmful toxins and restores the fragile balance of acidity and alkalinity in the body's internal chemistry.

The central tenet of food-combining is that protein foods, such as meat or beans, and starchy ones, such as potatoes or rice, are incompatible: eating them in a single meal is thought to wreak havoc with the digestive system and prevent the proper absorption of nutrients. Therefore, a stew that incorporated meat and potatoes, a breakfast of cereal and milk, or a sandwich pairing bread with cheese, meat, eggs or fish would be forbidden. The combination of grains and pulses, which are crucial sources of essential protein for vegans and vegetarians, would also be discouraged.

Other rules include banning fruit from meals and eating it only on its own as a separate meal or snack, and rejecting all processed foods. Taken literally, this rule would mean that even 100 per cent wholemeal bread baked from organic flours could not be consumed in the diet.

Scientists dismiss this system as a fad based on nutritional and physiological misconceptions. Most basic foods contain a combination of starches and proteins. The digestive tract does not distinguish between them, and the body is perfectly competent to process them when they arrive in the stomach at the same time.

The body also has its own internal mechanism for balancing acidity and alkalinity and for ridding itself of most naturally occurring toxins.

continued on page 138

The changing shape of women

Perceptions of the 'ideal' female shape have altered many times throughout the course of history.

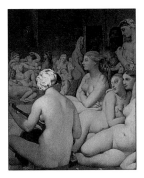

THE ROUNDED FIGURE
During the 18th century, an ample, curvy figure was often perceived by artists as representing female beauty.

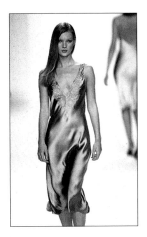

THE SLIM FIGURE
In the 20th century, perceptions of the ideal woman's body has ranged from the well-endowed Marilyn Monroe to the slender figure of the model Kate Moss.

135

The Dietitian

A dietitian's unique skill is to translate the science of nutrition into practical information about food. Dietitians advise people on dietary treatments for specific conditions, such as obesity or kidney disease, and about eating healthily.

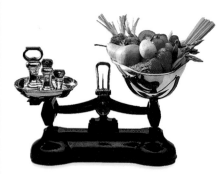

A QUESTION OF BALANCE
A dietitian will help you to achieve and maintain good health through a balanced diet that is personally tailored to meet your needs.

DETERMINING YOUR WEIGHT
If you decide that you want to lose weight, the dietitian will make a note of your weight and height in order to work out a realistic weight goal with you. He or she may also ask you to keep a food diary.

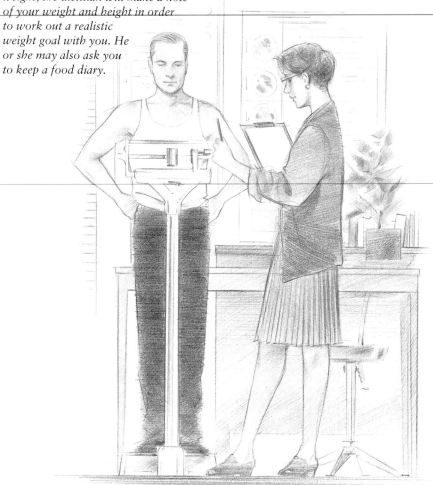

Degree-qualified and registered dietitians advise clients on their dietary needs. They often provide consultations at their own clinics but they may also work as part of a team, caring for people in a hospital or in the community. They work to a strict ethical code of conduct.

What is the difference between a nutritionist and a dietitian?
Although many nutritionists are qualified in nutrition, some may have undergone courses that are not recognised by academic or government bodies. Dietitians, on the other hand, have a degree in nutrition. Their studies in physiology and biochemistry lead to State Registration in Dietetics. The courses include a period of practical training in hospital and community settings, approved by the Dietitians' Board of the Council for Professions Supplementary to Medicine (CPSM).

Do I need a referral from my doctor to see a dietitian?
If you want general dietary assessment, weight control advice, healthy eating information or guidance on sports nutrition, no referral is necessary. But there are some disorders that require dietary treatment as part of their overall management, and for these you need a referral from a doctor or dentist. These conditions include: obesity and eating disorders; heart disease; food allergy; raised cholesterol; kidney and liver disease; coeliac disease; gastrointestinal disorders, such as irritable bowel syndrome, ulcerative colitis and constipation; and some cancers.

If I decide to lose weight, what will a dietitian ask me?
A dietitian will ask you about your current eating habits and lifestyle – for example, how often you eat, your

food likes and dislikes and whether you have any special dietary needs. You may be asked about your previous dieting experiences.

What do dietitians recommend as a healthy way to lose weight?

A dietitian will suggest that you follow a healthy balanced diet with a variety of foods. A recommended diet would aim at reducing your normal daily calorie intake by about 500 calories. For example, if you eat 2000 calories, you should reduce your intake to 1500 calories. (Women should not go below about 1200 calories a day and men should not go below about 1600 calories.)

Rather than count calories, the dietitian will help you to plan ways to lower your fat intake, particularly fried foods and fatty foods such as pastry, mayonnaise and biscuits. Keeping a food diary will help you to be more aware of your eating habits and give you a basis for making gradual changes. In addition, you will be encouraged to include regular exercise (for example, three to four times a week for 20 to 40 minutes or walking for two miles or more) to help maintain your metabolic rate and preserve or increase your lean tissue (muscle). Altogether the amount of weight you should lose is no more than 500 g to one kilogram (one to two pounds) per week, otherwise you will become too hungry and start losing lean tissue.

Will I need to take vitamin and mineral supplements?

A well-balanced diet should give you all the vitamins and minerals you need. It should be based on fresh fruit, vegetables, wholegrain cereals, low-fat protein foods and low-fat dairy products. Because it may be difficult to obtain enough iron, calcium, magnesium, zinc, riboflavin, B_6 and folic acid if your intake dips below 1200 to 1500 calories a day, the dietitian may advise, as a precaution, a multivitamin and mineral supplement to ensure that you are meeting your full nutrient

requirements. But aim to get as many of your vitamins and minerals as you can from your food first.

How often will I need to visit the dietitian to check my weight-loss progress?

Time between visits will vary from one to four weeks. Frequent appointments will help to keep you motivated. If you cannot manage regular appointments, ask your spouse or a friend to help check your weight and give you some encouragement. But your dietitian will be able to give you more detailed advice on each visit, talk over any of your specific dietary problems and discuss ways to help you to continue to improve your eating habits.

After I have reached the right weight, how long do I have to continue the weight-loss diet?

Once you have reached your healthy weight, you will be advised to gradually increase your calorie intake over

DIETITIAN'S KITCHEN TIPS

Here are some suggestions for reducing the amount of fat in your diet.

▶ *Thicken soups with 1 tablespoon of oatmeal instead of cream. The oatmeal adds extra fibre and vitamins.*

▶ *When making cakes, substitute a mashed banana for a third of the fat. You will achieve an equally good moist texture while dramatically reducing the fat content of the cake.*

a period of one to two weeks by eating larger quantities of low-fat, high-carbohydrate foods, for example, pasta. If you have made gradual and practical changes, you will find it easy not to revert to your old eating habits. Continue to eat the same well-balanced meals that you did when you were slimming and check your weight about every two weeks.

WHAT YOU CAN DO AT HOME

Most people who genuinely want to control their weight will take enough positive steps towards improvement. But there is little merit in trying to change old eating patterns overnight, sweeping everything from butter to

sausages to chocolate biscuits out of your life and kitchen forever, in a single, irrevocable act. The most effective changes are the ones that you make gradually – they may soon become just a habit.

1 *Eat less: butter, margarine and mayonnaise on sandwiches; fried foods like chips and doughnuts; fatty meats and meat products, for example burgers, sausages, luncheon meats and pork pies; pies and tarts; cakes, biscuits and puddings; chocolate; crisps and other snacks.*

2 *Change to lower-fat alternatives: skimmed or semi-skimmed milk instead of full fat; poultry (without skin) and the white meat rather than the dark; fish instead of red meat; trimmed lean meat instead of marbled; low-fat cheeses, such as cottage cheese, instead of hard cheese; grilled, stir-fried or baked food instead of fried or roasted food.*

MAKING A CHICKEN LEG LESS FATTY Chicken skin contains a lot of saturated fat so remove it before cooking. Using a pair of scissors, snip the edge of the chicken skin, then pull the chicken skin away from the meat.

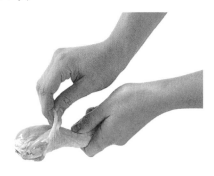

Can food burn fat?

There are even diets that tout the weight-reducing powers of particular foods. Nutritionists tend to dismiss these as fad or folklore.

Grapefruit, for instance, has often been promoted as a dieter's best friend, on the grounds that the acid or the enzymes within this fruit literally burn up body fat. With its high vitamin C content, grapefruit, like all fruit, is a valuable addition to any diet. But the notion that it can cut through fat in the same way that detergents cut through grease is simply erroneous.

HIDDEN FATS IN YOUR FOOD

Cutting down on excess fat and calories becomes much easier once you know where the hidden fats are lurking. It is important, therefore, to analyse the components of individual dishes to see how much fat they really contain.

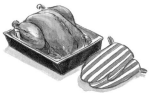

ROAST CHICKEN
Sixty-two per cent of the calories in a serving of roast chicken comes from the fat in the skin.

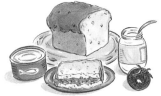

TUNA SANDWICH
Just over half the calories in a tuna, tomato and mayonnaise sandwich come from the fat in the mayonnaise.

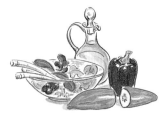

DRESSED SALAD
Ninety per cent of the calories in a green salad tossed with an oily or creamy dressing comes from the fat in the dressing rather than from the salad greens.

Not all popular diet systems deserve outright rejection. Any plan that features a healthy balance of different types of food, emphasises the consumption of fresh fruits, vegetables and grains, and encourages a reduced intake of calories and saturated fats is conveying a helpful message about healthy eating.

HARMING THE BODY

Certain diets, however, are not only lacking in benefits to health but may actively endanger it. Liquid diet formulas, for instance, if they are substituted for all or most regular meals, deliver speedy weight loss but ultimately are harmful to the body. They tend to be extremely low in calories – some provide no more than 300 to 500 calories per day – but excessively high in protein. A person sticking exclusively to such a diet will lose weight, but will simultaneously upset the balance of his or her endocrine system. The production of some essential hormones will be diminished, which can cause a variety of unpleasant symptoms ranging from constipation and abdominal bloating to nausea, dizziness and fatigue. Studies reveal that people who try these diets do lose weight but almost inevitably regain it.

For some dieters the health risk is even greater. A sudden switch away from this type of regime and back to a normal diet could result in a rapid drop in the levels of potassium and magnesium in the blood.

These minerals help to maintain the heart's normal rhythm, and in rare cases, such a disturbance could be fatal.

Fasting – literally starving to lose weight – is a very dangerous practice. If the body is not supplied with nutrients, it will exhaust its stores of fat then begin to digest its own muscles – including cardiac muscle, which can lead to heart failure. Other risks include gout and vitamin deficiency illnesses.

All crash diets have their perils. Bones can be weakened through lack of minerals, and nutritional imbalances may lead to the development of gallstones or even heart disease. Finally, these efforts interfere with the body's own normal weight-control mechanisms, with the result that any weight lost in this manner is likely to be regained faster and more easily than it would have been if no crash diet had ever been attempted.

The only safe, healthy and reliable way to lose weight is to do it slowly and gradually, with a permanent adjustment of eating habits, accompanied by an increase in energy expenditure through regular exercise.

The fashionable body

Many of the people who attempt a weight-reduction diet do not, in fact, need to lose weight. Women especially suffer from the modern Western cultural obsession with a slim, boyish, willowy figure. They often believe themselves to be overweight when by any medical standards they are not.

Skeletal fashion models parade down the catwalks. Film actresses who are anything other than slim virtually never play romantic heroines. The clothes on sale in many modish shops are available only in sizes that exclude virtually half the female population, as are those portrayed in fashion magazines.

For many individuals, but especially for emotionally vulnerable adolescent girls, this cult of fanatical slenderness combines with psychological problems such as low self-esteem, in the development of potentially life-threatening eating disorders, such as anorexia nervosa. Anorexics believe themselves to be fat, even when they are visibly emaciated, and deliberately starve to get even thinner. Long-term effects of the illness include a damaged immune system, anaemia, osteoporosis and heart disease. Another eating disorder, bulimia, leads to a pattern of alternately bingeing on food and equally compulsive self-induced vomiting, starvation or massive consumption of laxatives.

There are, indeed, many adults – and children – in the affluent Western world who are to some degree overweight, even obese. And because of sedentary lifestyles and unhealthy diets, the number continues to rise. British figures for 1994, for instance, indicated that the rates of obesity had more than doubled in six years – 13 per cent of men and 16 per cent of women were obese.

A moderate amount of excess poundage is not the same as obesity, and it is important to distinguish between the two.

CHANGING HABITS

A substantial amount of calories can be eliminated by reviewing everyday eating habits. Change to low-fat milk, preferably skimmed. Use salad dressings sparingly, or make your own with extra vinegar and less oil. Replace fried potatoes with baked or boiled ones and eat crisps only as a special treat, if ever. Increase the number of servings of fruit and vegetables and avoid all sauces on them. Reduce the size of servings of meat and poultry and replace them with eggs, fish or pulses for a few meals each week. Serve salads as a starter and, where possible, use low-fat cheeses. Cut out high-fat drinks, desserts and snacks, and watch what you put on your bread.

Dried fruits have a role in healthy eating, although they are high in sugar and so cannot be eaten with quite the same freedom as the fresh varieties. An unsweetened breakfast cereal, for instance, is tastier with a sprinkling of raisins or other chopped dried fruit. The fruit supplies not only sweetness, but fibre, vitamins and minerals. Since even a 30 gram (one ounce) serving of conventionally sweetened commercial breakfast cereal may contain as many as four teaspoons of sugar, it is highly preferable to 'sweeten' a serving of unsweetened breakfast cereal with the extra nutrition that even a few raisins can add.

For many people the idea of eliminating certain treat foods – ice cream, for example, or chocolate – drives them to guilty binges on these very same foods. But by allowing one modest and carefully rationed indulgence every day – a single sweet biscuit or a few spoonfuls of ice cream – it is possible to curb any desperate cravings. Give yourself an allowance of pleasurable foods every day, but limit this to one treat only – a croissant for breakfast, a biscuit after lunch or ice cream at dinner – but not all three.

continued on page 142

DO YOU NEED TO LOSE WEIGHT?

One simple indicator of excess body fat is the waist-hip ratio, which shows the presence of fat on the abdomen.

For women, a ratio higher than 0.8 indicates that there is excessive abdominal fat. For men, the crucial maximum is 0.95. If your ratio is higher than this, you may be well advised to lose weight. In a society obsessed with slim figures, an individual may feel pressured to lose weight even when he or she is well within the range considered healthy for his or her age and size.

1 *To measure your waist-hip ratio, use a tape measure to find out the circumference of your waist, including any protruding stomach.*

2 *Repeat the above process to measure the circumference of your hips.*

3 *Divide the measurement of the waist by the hip measurement. The result is your waist-hip ratio.*

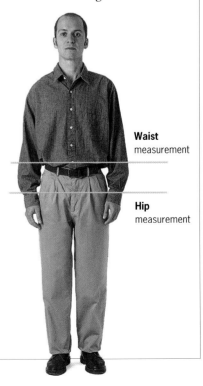

Waist
measurement

Hip
measurement

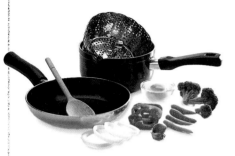

Cooking for a

Low-fat Diet

For those who genuinely want to control their weight or improve their general health, the surest path to success lies in the ability to make basic, and permanent, changes in eating habits and attitudes.

ESSENTIAL UTENSILS
Non-stick pots and pans radically reduce the amount of cooking oil needed for sautéing meats and vegetables, making pancakes and omelettes and reheating cooked food.

For successful dieting, you require both a combination of nutritional knowledge and self-discipline. You need to know which foods are fattening and have a sound sense of caloric content as well as portion size control.

To stay healthy and well-nourished, you should eat a wide variety of fresh foods in well-balanced combinations.

This type of eating pattern will help you to avoid an excess of those elements, like saturated fats, that are detrimental both to your health and to the success of your diet.

It also helps, strange as it may seem, to enjoy good food, to plan meals creatively and to look forward to them as a source not just of nourishment but of positive pleasure.

MAKING THE RIGHT CUTS

Before cooking fatty cuts of meat, such as lamb or pork chops, remove the external fat.

LIGHTLY DOES IT

A considerable saving of fat calories can be made by a slight adjustment to normal preparation and cooking

techniques. Even when you are using ordinary cookware, you can cut down on your use of oil.

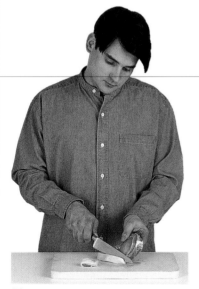

TRIMMING FAT
Using a sharp knife, trim off excess fat from around the chop. Do not remove all the fat, however, or the chop will lose its shape and moisture when cooked.

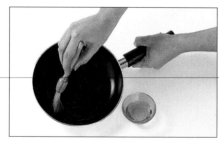

OILING WITH A BRUSH
Instead of pouring oil from the bottle straight into the frying pan, use an oil-dipped pastry brush or kitchen paper to apply a much lighter coating.

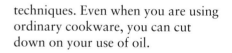
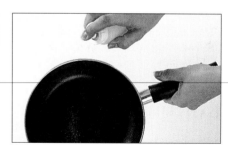

OILING WITH SPRAY
For a very fine coating of oil, use a non-aerosol oil spray. Hold the spray 15 cm (6 in) from the pan and give two to three squirts. Do not use near flame.

CHOOSING LEAN MEAT

When you want to eat meat, you can save many fat calories even before you start to cook by selecting the least fatty cuts.

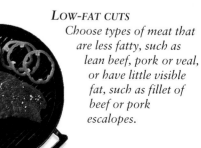

LOW-FAT CUTS
Choose types of meat that are less fatty, such as lean beef, pork or veal, or have little visible fat, such as fillet of beef or pork escalopes.

CUTTING BACK ON OIL

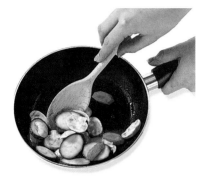

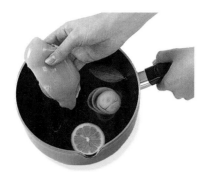

Spoon off
and discard
excess fat

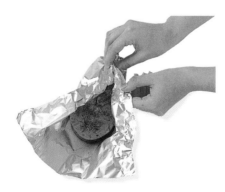

JUICE OR STOCK ALTERNATIVES
You can sauté some foods successfully by replacing the oil with a nonfat cooking liquid. Try simmering vegetables in tomato juice or fresh chicken stock that has been skimmed of all fat.

POACHING
Cook chicken or fish in a court bouillon – water acidulated with a little lemon juice or vinegar and seasoned with such herbs as fresh parsley, chervil and thyme.

SKIMMING FAT
Prepare stocks, stews, roasts and soups in advance and chill them for several hours or overnight. The fat within them will rise to the top and solidify and will be easy to remove. The same strategy can be applied when making meat or chicken broths.

STEAMING VEGETABLES

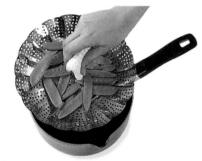

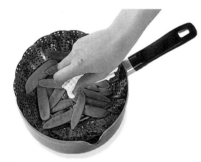

1 *A basket steamer that fits into a conventional saucepan is ideal for individual portions of vegetables. Keep the vegetables well-spaced in a single layer for even steaming.*

2 *Make sure the water in the saucepan is boiling before placing the basket steamer inside. There should be about 2.5 cm (1 in) of water to allow steaming, but it should not touch the vegetables.*

BAKING FISH IN FOIL

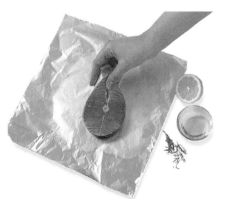

QUICK TIPS FOR LESS CHOLESTEROL

Here are a few ideas to help you reduce the amount of cholesterol in your diet.

▶ *Top a baked potato with low-fat cottage cheese and chives.*

▶ *Instead of sautéing mushrooms in butter, cook them in a little Worcestershire sauce.*

▶ *Experiment with interesting continental and wholegrain breads, for example, rye bread with caraway seeds; they are so rich in flavour that they do not need to be spread with butter or mayonnaise.*

▶ *Instead of covering baked vegetable dishes with grated cheese, top with fresh wholemeal breadcrumbs seasoned with herbs and drizzle a thimbleful of olive oil over the crumbs. Brown for a few minutes under the grill to form a light, crispy topping.*

▶ *Purée cooked pulses to make a thick-textured soup without using cream or a roux-based sauce.*

▶ *Thicken sauces with vegetable purées, or use the purée as a sauce.*

▶ *When making burgers, make them with half minced beef and half minced turkey.*

1 *A good alternative to frying fish is to bake it in aluminium foil. Lightly oil a square of foil and place the fish in the centre. Sprinkle with lemon juice and fresh herbs such as dill.*

2 *Pull the edges of the foil up to cover the fish. Pinch the foil parcel together to seal, then bake. Alternatively, wrap the fish in baking parchment. Proceed as for foil but fold over the edges.*

Fast-food choices

A fast-food restaurant does not have to be a dietary disaster area. Some chains, aware of the commercial advantage to be gained by catering to the growing number of weight-conscious consumers, now provide salad selections or special 'healthy option' sections on their menus.

Even where choice is limited, it is possible to avoid excessive fat intake by choosing grilled chicken on a bun instead of chicken nuggets coated in batter and deep-fried or opting for a plain beefburger dressed with a little mustard or ketchup instead of one topped with melted cheese.

EATING OUT AND WATCHING YOUR WEIGHT

If all meals were eaten at home, then weight control would be much easier. But many people find the hardest part of maintaining a reasonable diet is when eating in restaurants. When dining out, the restaurant you choose may make a vital difference in your ability to maintain your diet. A restaurant with an all-you-can-eat set-price buffet may be a good buy, but avoid it unless you are sure that some of the items on the heavily laden board are genuinely low-fat options.

Steakhouses famous for their giant cuts of marbled prime beef are equally unsuitable for anyone who wants to lose weight, as are old-fashioned restaurants specialising in the traditional butter-and-cream-based grande cuisine. In a large town or city, with many different cuisines available, the best course of action may be to choose a restaurant that serves food from a region or country known for its healthy diet.

In a Chinese or Japanese restaurant, for instance, a diligent diner will find a wide selection of healthy, low-fat dishes: lightly cooked fresh fish; steamed rice topped with stir-fried vegetables and lean, slivered poultry; and light and crunchy salads. Italian restaurants can be another good choice, as long as heavily creamed pasta sauces are avoided in favour of tomato-based varieties, or if the pasta is tossed in a little olive oil and garlic and herbs. (And if you use the Parmesan cheese sparingly.) Restaurants that specialise in seafood are another good source of healthy options, but choose dishes that are grilled or steamed, not deep-fried.

Any type of establishment worth a visit should be able to accommodate the needs of weight-conscious customers. If booking in advance, ask whether the menu includes any low-fat dishes or if the chef is willing, with a bit of notice, to prepare a dish with just a minimum of fat. In restaurants where all the food is cooked to order there should be no difficulty in meeting special requests, such as having for an accompanying sauce served on the side so that you can control the quantity that you use.

Many misguided diners-out imagine that they can save calories in advance by skipping lunch or starving themselves on the day of a restaurant dinner. In fact, the hungrier you are, the more likely you are to order – and consume – too much food or succumb to the richest temptations on the menu. One useful tactic is to eat a piece of fruit or some other low-fat snack just before leaving home. Then, when you arrive at the restaurant, you will not feel ravenous; instead you will be ready to enjoy your meal.

EATING OUT: SLIMMER'S SURVIVAL TIPS

You do not have to give up all your social activities when trying to control your weight. Use the following tips to guide you through the high-calorie maze of dining out in restaurants.

▶ *Avoid 'money-saving' fixed-price multi-course dinners. What you save in money you may pay for in excess calories. Choose from the à la carte menu, even if the individual dishes cost a little more, and limit yourself to the amount of food you really need.*

▶ *Bear in mind that you do not have to eat all the food on your plate. If the portion is large you can ask the waiter to have your meal divided in two and have one half parcelled up for you to take home. Most restaurants are happy to cooperate.*

▶ *Do not choose your dessert until you have finished eating your main course: you will make a far more sensible choice than you would on an empty stomach.*

A LITTLE ON THE SIDE
Order your side salad either with the dressing on the side or with cruets of vinegar and olive oil. Then you can dress the salad sparingly or with only a touch of oil. Most kitchens are over generous with high-fat dressings.

CHAPTER 9

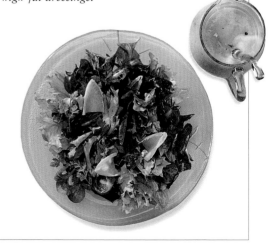

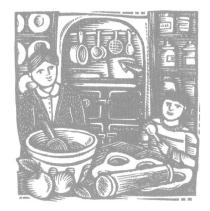

A HEALTHY KITCHEN

*It is easy to forget, during the daily
chore of providing meals for all the family,
that food can be one of the great pleasures in life.
To make the most of food, however, it needs to be
properly prepared, cooked and stored; otherwise
vital nutrients will be lost or individuals may be put
at risk from food poisoning. Safe and healthy
cooking techniques can safeguard your
health and that of your family.*

THE RAW MATERIALS

To get the most from your foods you should be aware of how to buy and store them so that they maintain their quality and are completely safe from contamination.

CHILLED FOODS

Developing good habits for safely refrigerating food is easy. Follow the tips below to help prevent food poisoning.

▶ *Refrigerate food as soon as possible. Cover or wrap all food and never use unwashed containers. Do not reuse old cling film, plastic bags, paper wrappings or foil with fresh or frozen food.*

▶ *When thawing frozen foods, make sure that liquid does not drip onto other food. The blood of raw meat should never be allowed to drip onto other foods because it is a major cause of food poisoning. Wrap it carefully and place meat on the lower shelves.*

▶ *Check the 'use-by' date. If the food is not dated and you cannot remember when it was refrigerated, then throw it away.*

Cleanliness and proper food handling are of primary concern in the kitchen because bacteria can multiply in its warm atmosphere at a prodigious rate, bringing with them the peril of food poisoning. The goal of kitchen hygiene is to reduce this risk to zero by giving bacteria as little opportunity for growth as possible.

Keep cold food in the refrigerator until it is ready to be served; all hot food should be thoroughly cooked to ensure all bacteria are killed. This particularly applies to whole poultry and meats, especially burgers and rolled roasts because bacteria can lurk in the centre of these foods. If you have to delay serving hot food, make sure that it has been thoroughly cooked first to kill off

bacteria and then keep it very hot, above 60°C (140°F). If the food is left standing below this temperature, bacteria will start to develop again. Food poisoning bacteria will also survive in food that has not been cooked through. Use a cooking or meat thermometer to check the food's temperature. Be careful not to let the thermometer touch the bottom of the pan or it will give the wrong reading.

ROOM TEMPERATURE

Bacteria grow rapidly and produce toxins in temperatures between 16°C and 60°C (61°F and 140°F). Therefore, do not allow cooked foods to be left at room temperature for more than two hours. The warmer the

---

CLEANLINESS IN THE KITCHEN

Scrupulous hygiene is the key to a safe kitchen, but this is not as daunting as it sounds. The aim is not sterile operating-theatre standards but basic domestic hygiene. To achieve this, follow the steps outlined below.

▶ *Wash your hands with warm water and soap before preparing food, and clean all work surfaces daily using a disinfectant designed for food preparation areas.*

▶ *Wipe surfaces dry, as moisture provides a potential breeding ground for bacteria.*

▶ *Do not place cooked or ready-to-eat food on a surface that has had raw food on it unless you clean it thoroughly first. Raw food, particularly poultry, meat and fish, is more likely to have bacteria on it, which will transfer to the cooked food.*

▶ *Wipe up food spills as they occur using a clean cloth or kitchen paper. Use kitchen paper to mop up spills on the kitchen floor.*

▶ *After use, leave kitchen cloths to soak in a mild bleach solution, and change tea towels every day to prevent bacteria from building up and contaminating surfaces with which the cloths come into contact.*

▶ *Whether you use an acrylic chopping board or a wooden one, you should pour boiling water over the board to sterilise it or soak it in a mild bleach solution for a minute. Rinse with clean water.*

CHOPPING SAFELY
Clean your knife and board thoroughly after chopping meat and before chopping vegetables.

temperature of the room, the shorter the time that cooked food should be left standing. If the room's temperature is 32°C (90°F) or higher, do not leave the food out for more than an hour, and preferably not at all.

Throw away any dairy, egg, meat, poultry or fish dishes that have been left at room temperature for more than two hours. After storing leftover food in the refrigerator or freezer, reheat it at no less than 74°C (165°F) and serve while it is still hot.

REFRIGERATION

All perishable foods should be stored in the refrigerator. These foods include meat, fish, poultry and dairy products, as well as salads and leafy green vegetables. Use different parts of the refrigerator for the various foods. Keep raw meat, bacon, poultry and fish in the coldest part of the refrigerator – usually the bottom shelf. Put cooked dishes on the centre shelves, and vegetables and salads in the salad drawer. Ideally, dairy products should be stored in the door of the refrigerator, because it is often cooler than the top shelves in the cabinet area. Root vegetables such as carrots can be stored in a cool cupboard but will also keep well in the refrigerator. Avoid overfilling the refrigerator because this blocks the circulation of air.

For maximum efficiency, the temperature of the refrigerator should be between 0°C and 5°C (32°F and 41°F). Keep a refrigerator thermometer in the coldest section and try to check the temperature every day.

Before cleaning the refrigerator, remove all the foods and cover them with a clean sheet or newspapers to keep them cool. Clean the refrigerator with a recommended cleaner or wipe surfaces with a solution of bicarbonate of soda and warm water. Household soaps and detergents may leave behind a smell that will taint the food.

FREEZER SAFETY

The low temperature of the freezer preserves the food and prevents nutritional loss by arresting bacterial activity that starts the decay. Freezers should be set at -18°C (0°F) or below for rapid freezing.

Overwrap packages for freezing in freezer wrap or bags or with aluminium foil. Before freezing cooked foods, place them in airtight containers about eight centimetres (three inches) high or less, leaving some space for expansion, and make sure they are tightly closed. If foods are refrigerated or frozen in large, deep containers, the food in the middle stays warm longer and bacteria can grow in this area. Label packages with the contents and date. Most foods can be frozen safely providing they are well wrapped. But a few foods should not be frozen: eggs in their shells will crack and milk may separate.

Many foods – for example soup and most vegetables – can be cooked without thawing first, but other foods need to be thoroughly

CONTROLLING HOUSEHOLD PESTS

The kitchen is a breeding ground for pests, which enter uninvited and damage cupboard contents, infect food and spread disease. All pests need to be evicted. This chart shows what to do.

RECOGNISING SIGNS	WHAT TO DO
ANTS	
Columns of ants marching to and from the nest, or inside the house.	Puff ant killer into the nest and along route of entry to the house.
MICE	
Evidence of droppings; packets of food chewed and contents spilt.	Use a mousetrap. For infestations, use an approved chemical substance (follow instructions carefully).
RATS	
Loud, pronounced gnawing; large holes in packets of food, and even nonfood items, such as curtains.	Contact your local environmental health department or a pest control expert. Do not leave lids off outside bins.
FLIES	
Maggots; loud buzzing; most prevalent in hot, humid weather and when food is left uncovered.	Use fly sprays or strips containing a contact insecticide. Make sure bins are cleared daily.
COCKROACHES	
Tiny dots of droppings concentrated around areas such as drawers and tiny gaps where they hide during the day.	Detector traps are available – a sticky pad with hormone attractant. Use insecticide or contact a pest control expert.
MITES	
Almost invisible, mites resemble moving dust particles and infest flour, cereals, rice and pasta that have become damp.	Dispose of affected food. Wash out cupboards with a disinfectant and store the replacement foods in sealed containers.

defrosted beforehand, especially large pieces of meat and meat sauces. Defrosting ensures that the centre of the food is properly cooked. Thaw foods in the refrigerator, in the microwave, or in cold water, but not at room temperature. When defrosting the freezer, wrap food in clean newspaper to prevent it thawing before refreezing.

CHOOSING FRESH FOODS

When choosing fresh food, rely on your senses of touch, sight, smell and taste. If you are in any doubt, do not buy it. Only buy foods from reputable sources and avoid bargains unless you intend to eat them on the day of purchase. Always take notice of the 'use-by' or 'best before' dates for dairy

CHECKING FOOD QUALITY

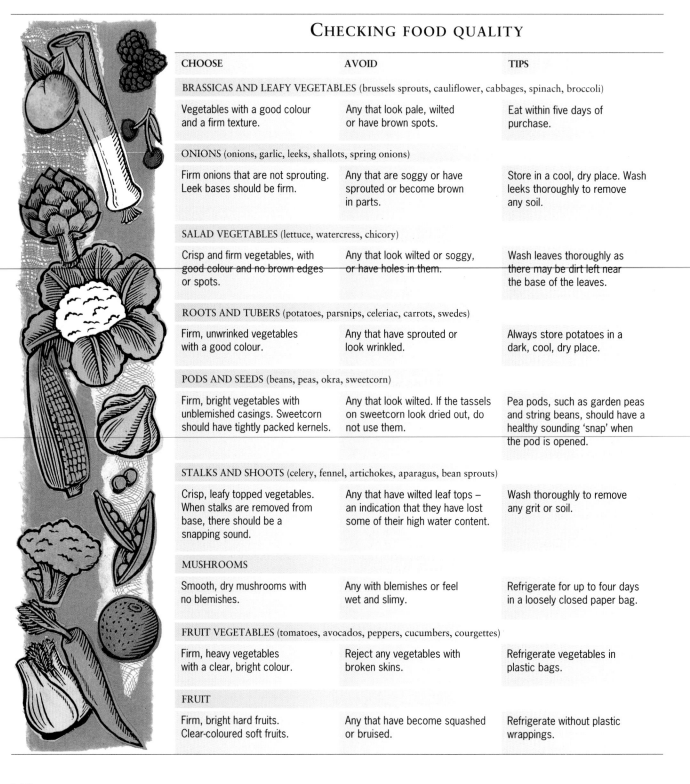

CHOOSE	AVOID	TIPS
BRASSICAS AND LEAFY VEGETABLES (brussels sprouts, cauliflower, cabbages, spinach, broccoli)		
Vegetables with a good colour and a firm texture.	Any that look pale, wilted or have brown spots.	Eat within five days of purchase.
ONIONS (onions, garlic, leeks, shallots, spring onions)		
Firm onions that are not sprouting. Leek bases should be firm.	Any that are soggy or have sprouted or become brown in parts.	Store in a cool, dry place. Wash leeks thoroughly to remove any soil.
SALAD VEGETABLES (lettuce, watercress, chicory)		
Crisp and firm vegetables, with good colour and no brown edges or spots.	Any that look wilted or soggy, or have holes in them.	Wash leaves thoroughly as there may be dirt left near the base of the leaves.
ROOTS AND TUBERS (potatoes, parsnips, celeriac, carrots, swedes)		
Firm, unwrinkled vegetables with a good colour.	Any that have sprouted or look wrinkled.	Always store potatoes in a dark, cool, dry place.
PODS AND SEEDS (beans, peas, okra, sweetcorn)		
Firm, bright vegetables with unblemished casings. Sweetcorn should have tightly packed kernels.	Any that look wilted. If the tassels on sweetcorn look dried out, do not use them.	Pea pods, such as garden peas and string beans, should have a healthy sounding 'snap' when the pod is opened.
STALKS AND SHOOTS (celery, fennel, artichokes, aparagus, bean sprouts)		
Crisp, leafy topped vegetables. When stalks are removed from base, there should be a snapping sound.	Any that have wilted leaf tops – an indication that they have lost some of their high water content.	Wash thoroughly to remove any grit or soil.
MUSHROOMS		
Smooth, dry mushrooms with no blemishes.	Any with blemishes or feel wet and slimy.	Refrigerate for up to four days in a loosely closed paper bag.
FRUIT VEGETABLES (tomatoes, avocados, peppers, cucumbers, courgettes)		
Firm, heavy vegetables with a clear, bright colour.	Reject any vegetables with broken skins.	Refrigerate vegetables in plastic bags.
FRUIT		
Firm, bright hard fruits. Clear-coloured soft fruits.	Any that have become squashed or bruised.	Refrigerate without plastic wrappings.

products, meats and processed foods, and be ruthless about discarding food that has passed its peak. Buy fruits and vegetables often, preferably every two to three days.

When choosing seafood, the old maxim that you should eat shellfish only during the months that contain the letter *r*: from September to April, can be of use. There are several types of shellfish caught or farmed in British waters. Most are available throughout the year, but some, such as the European oyster, cannot be eaten during the breeding season (May to August) because of poor quality. Crabs and lobsters sometimes hibernate in cold water so are more abundant from April to October. Scallops are usually

CHECKING FOOD QUALITY

CHOOSE	AVOID	TIPS
RED MEAT		
Beef with a deep red colour and creamy coloured fat. Pork should be pale pink with a close-grained texture and an even covering of fat. Choose plump joints of lamb with pliable skin and creamy coloured fat.	Beef that has an unnatural bright orange colour or any pork with a greyish tinge and an oily fat covering. Avoid lamb with fat that is yellow and oily – this indicates an older piece of meat.	Beef, pork and lamb can be kept for up to three days in the refrigerator. Pork can be kept for up to eight months and beef and lamb for up to a year in the freezer.
POULTRY		
Birds with a plump, well-rounded breast and skin that is firm and slightly creamy yellow in colour.	Any bird that looks underfed and that has blemishes and bruises on its skin. Also avoid frozen birds that have frozen moisture in the package – this indicates they have thawed and been refrozen.	Refrigerate for up to two days and freeze for up to six months. Frozen birds must be defrosted thoroughly before cooking.
FISH		
Only the freshest fish. Choose from a reputable fishmonger or supermarket and eat on the day of purchase. Fish should smell of the sea and have plenty of scales, and bright eyes. The gills should be red and the flesh firm. Frozen fish should be frozen solid with no signs of water.	Any fish that has a strong fishy smell – an indication of high levels of bacteria – or dull, opaque eyes. Also avoid fish with slimy skin (although some fresh water fish have slime on them). The flesh of fresh fish bounces back immediately when pressed.	Fish should be refrigerated for only one day – in the coldest section – and frozen for up to six months. Oily fish spoils more easily: freeze for up to three months only. Fish that is bought frozen can be kept in the freezer and defrosted or cooked from frozen.
SHELLFISH		
Live mussels and oysters should have tightly closed shells or, if opened, should close when tapped. Raw and cooked prawns should be firm. Judge cooked lobsters and crabs by weight as well as size – good ones should feel heavy for their size.	Mussels, clams and oysters that are open before cooking or that have failed to open after cooking. Avoid any shellfish with cracked or chipped shells. Do not buy, eat or serve any shellfish that is more than a day old.	Raw or cooked prawns and cooked mussels can be frozen for up to a month. Cooked crab and lobster meat can be frozen for up to two months.
DAIRY PRODUCE AND EGGS		
Products with a good, clear colour and a fresh smell. Do not take any chances, particularly with eggs.	Cheese, butter or milk that smells sour or rancid, and milk that has separated and looks watery. Do not buy eggs that are cracked.	Eggs should last two weeks from purchase. Milk should be stored for up to four days only. Hard cheese can be refrigerated for up to a few months, soft cheese for only a week or two.

eaten during the summer months, but the mussel season is normally between September and March, when their meat is most plump.

STORING FOOD IN THE CUPBOARD
When the unexpected happens – visitors, illness or bad weather – a well-stocked store cupboard will help you to provide delicious, nourishing meals. The foods in your larder are reliable standbys because they have long shelf lives. No food lasts forever, however, and over time, food stored in the larder is just as susceptible to contamination and infestation as other foods. Every few days, check your cupboard and throw away any product that has exceeded its 'use-by' date.

FOODS FOR THE CUPBOARD SHELF

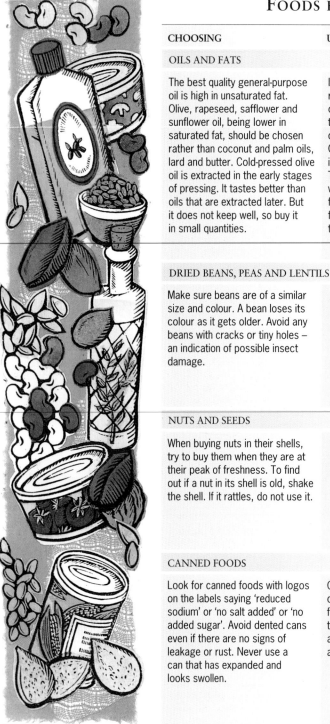

CHOOSING	USING	STORING
OILS AND FATS		
The best quality general-purpose oil is high in unsaturated fat. Olive, rapeseed, safflower and sunflower oil, being lower in saturated fat, should be chosen rather than coconut and palm oils, lard and butter. Cold-pressed olive oil is extracted in the early stages of pressing. It tastes better than oils that are extracted later. But it does not keep well, so buy it in small quantities.	If you must deep-fry, use oil rather than fat and only use the oil once. Deep-frying changes the oil because food fried in it dissolves its fat into the oil. Gradual oxidation occurs, which is the early stage of rancidity. The oil will become darker and will foam on the surface when food is added. Also, reusing oil for deep-frying causes vitamin E to be lost.	Never mix used oil with new. Oils may go rancid, smelling and tasting stale, when they should be thrown away. When used oil is cold, it may congeal. If this happens, it will liquefy when brought back to room temperature. Unopened oil in glass bottles will keep for many months provided you store it in a dark, cool place. Once opened, oils usually last for about six months.
DRIED BEANS, PEAS AND LENTILS		
Make sure beans are of a similar size and colour. A bean loses its colour as it gets older. Avoid any beans with cracks or tiny holes – an indication of possible insect damage.	Before cooking, pick over the beans or peas and discard any stones or grit. Most beans need to be soaked for about eight hours before cooking and boiled in fresh water for 10 minutes to eliminate toxins. Follow packet instructions.	Because they contain almost no fat, dried beans (except soya beans, which are high in fat) are ideal for storing in the cupboard, but they should be eaten within a year. Store in an airtight container in a cool, dry place.
NUTS AND SEEDS		
When buying nuts in their shells, try to buy them when they are at their peak of freshness. To find out if a nut in its shell is old, shake the shell. If it rattles, do not use it.	Most shelled nuts can be bought whole, chopped, ground or blanched and require no preparation.	Both nuts and seeds should be stored in a cool, dry place to preserve their oil content as long as possible. Store shelled nuts in airtight containers in the refrigerator. The shop packaging is not ideal for long-term storage.
CANNED FOODS		
Look for canned foods with logos on the labels saying 'reduced sodium' or 'no salt added' or 'no added sugar'. Avoid dented cans even if there are no signs of leakage or rust. Never use a can that has expanded and looks swollen.	Once opened, the contents will deteriorate at the same rate as fresh cooked food. Never keep the contents in an open can, as this could lead to metal absorption.	Cans can be stored for four to five years but check the 'use-by' date. If a can becomes rusty, dented or has expanded, throw it away, as the food inside may be contaminated. Botulism – a form of food poisoning – can occur through home canning if rules for canning methods and hygiene are not followed.

Also pay attention to 'best-before' dates, which show only the month and year for products that last longer than three months.

When stocking the cupboard with new foods, use a rotation system. Move the older foods forward and place the new ones behind them so that the old foods are eaten first. Whenever you do this, make sure that you throw away any foods that are growing mould and any cans that have expanded or become rusty. To avoid insect infestations and contamination of food, clean out the store cupboard regularly with a mild disinfectant. Preferably use a brand specifically made for food surfaces so that there will be no danger of tainting the food.

FOODS FOR THE CUPBOARD SHELF

CHOOSING	USING	STORING
BREAKFAST CEREALS		
Choose cereals with a high fibre content. Avoid cartons that are torn or show signs of leakage. Sometimes they are accidentally slit by the store stacker opening the case with a sharp knife.	Instead of sugar, sprinkle pieces of chopped fruit, such as bananas, or dried fruit, such as raisins, onto the cereal.	Once opened, seal packets with food clips or fold over the inner lining of the packet. Store the box in a cool, dry place.
PASTA AND NOODLES		
Dried pasta and noodles should be brittle and smooth. Choose pasta made from wholemeal flour, which contains more fibre and zinc than refined flour.	Pasta and noodles require no preparation before cooking. Allow 115 g (4 oz) of uncooked pasta per person and cook until 'al dente' (offering some resistance to the teeth).	Dried pasta and noodles have a long shelf life when correctly stored because microorganisms rarely grow on them. Store them in an airtight container in a cool, dry place. Do not let them become exposed to moisture.
FLOUR		
Some of the vitamins and minerals lost in the refining process are replaced in white flour by manufacturers, but it lacks fibre. Wholemeal flour contains about 10.8 g fibre per 100 g (3½ oz) of flour. Avoid any packets that are torn or show signs of leakage.	Pass the flour through a sieve to remove any lumps. If a recipe specifies sifting before using, be sure to follow the directions.	Keep the flour in a cool, dry cupboard in an airtight container. Flour is vulnerable to insects – flour mites, weevils, moths and beetles – so check regularly and discard the flour if you find any. You will have to wash down the cupboard with a mild disinfectant and scrupulously clean the container the flour was kept in.
HERBS		
Only buy small amounts of dried herbs, as they will lose their pungency and flavour after a few months.	Dried herbs require no preparation before using. They are best used in slow-cooking dishes for a stronger flavour.	Keep dried herbs away from heat and light and store in airtight containers. Chopped fresh herbs can be frozen in ice-cube trays filled with water.
SPICES		
Buy spices whole whenever possible, as they will retain their flavour and freshness much better.	Grind whole spices using a pestle and mortar or electric coffee grinder. If using whole spices in stews or soups, wrap in a muslin bag and tie the string to the pan handle for easy removal.	Keep in airtight jars, away from light and moisture. Many spices have long shelf lives but keep an eye on the 'use-by' date and discard if exceeded, as they tend to taste dry and dusty.

COOKING FOR BETTER HEALTH

Cooking enhances the flavour, appearance, smell and texture of foods. But it is important to know which methods are best for preserving the nutritional content and promoting cooking safety.

Not only does food tend to look and taste better when it is prepared and cooked well, but the nutritional content is much more valuable, sometimes up to three times greater than that of badly cooked food. Overexposure to air, too much added fat, excessive heat, an unsuitable cooking method and other variables can destroy nutritional quality.

VEGETABLES

Both light and air as well as heat affect the nutritional content of vegetables. In order to preserve their goodness, do not wash, chop, slice or cook vegetables until you are ready to use them. Fruits and vegetables contain enzymes that cause them to ripen and lose nutrients. Since warm temperatures accelerate the enzyme activity, store fruits and vegetables in airtight containers in the refrigerator.

Wash vegetables before using, but do not soak them because water-soluble nutrients will leach into the water. Hold them briefly under cold running water and use a vegetable scrubbing brush to remove dirt from root vegetables like carrots.

Peeled vegetables are less nutritious as much of their nutritional content lies just beneath the surface of the skin. If you do not want to eat vegetables unpeeled, cook them in their skins, then it will be much easier to peel off their skins and fewer nutrients are lost.

Retaining nutrients

Avoid boiling vegetables because much of their nutritional goodness will disappear into the water. Instead, steam vegetables, cook them in a microwave, or stir-fry them using a minimum amount of water or oil. They should be cooked until 'al dente' (that is, they offer some resistance to the teeth, instead of being soft and soggy), so that they retain their colour and texture. Do not use bicarbonate of soda to preserve colour; alkaline solutions destroy vitamins.

MICROWAVE COOKING

Microwaves cook by making the water molecules in food vibrate quickly, and so generate heat. The microwaves penetrate to a depth of only one to two inches, so the heat spreads through the food by conduction – the food cooks from the outside inwards.

Microwave ovens are quick and efficient and use very little liquid for cooking. They are ideal for steaming fish and vegetables, which lose the minimum amount of nutrients. But foods cook unevenly and there are 'cold spots' and 'hot spots'. Using a rotating turntable and stirring will cook food more evenly. This also solves an important problem because food-poisoning bacteria may grow in a cold spot. Always observe 'standing' times after cooking because they are part of the overall cooking.

OVEN-BAKED POTATO
The hot, dry air in a conventional oven penetrates a potato slowly. After about 15 minutes the centre is still cool. It takes about an hour to cook through.

MICROWAVED POTATO
Although microwaving heats the potato through after about five minutes, standing time is needed for thorough cooking.

After 7 minutes　**After 15 minutes**

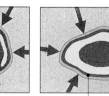

Heat slowly spreads through conduction

After 1¹/₂ minutes　**After 5 minutes**

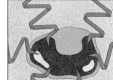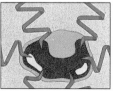

Vibrating molecules generate heat, which spreads through conduction

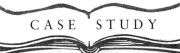

A Vegetarian in the Family

In a household where meat is the principal source of protein, the sudden decision of an adolescent son or daughter to switch to a vegetarian diet can throw the family cook into a quandary. Where will the teenager get the protein he or she needs for a healthy, well-balanced diet? And does this mean that every meal will require the preparation of two separate menus?

Sixteen-year-old Sarah, who is interested in environmental issues, announces to her parents that she has become a vegetarian. Her mother, Liz, is not entirely surprised. Although Liz is an enthusiastic cook with a large collection of recipe books, her meals have always been meat-oriented: beef and lamb stews, chops, and a traditional roast on Sundays. Food shopping routinely ends with a trip to the local delicatessen, for the pâtés, salamis and hams that the family favours for sandwiches and snacks. And, although she wants to keep Sarah happy, Liz cannot take on too much extra catering: she teaches at a primary school, and is studying part-time for a degree.

WHAT SHOULD LIZ DO?

Liz should start by investigating nonmeat sources of protein and iron to make sure that Sarah does not suffer deficiencies in her diet. Once she explores her local health food shop and scans a few vegetarian cookery books, she will be reassured about the wide range of alternative protein sources. Not only the predictable options of dairy products but combinations of grains and pulses that provide as much protein as one of her husband's steaks. If she does not object to convenience foods, she can buy a wide selection of pies based on tofu or pulses and meatless sausages made with textured vegetable protein, known as TVP.

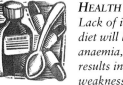

HEALTH
Lack of iron in the diet will lead to anaemia, which results in tiredness, weakness and breathlessness.

A VARIED DIET
If a vegetarian diet is not well thought out, it may become as unbalanced as that of many meat eaters.

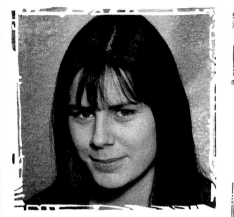

COOKING METHODS
Many vegetarian dishes take longer to prepare if made from scratch.

Action Plan

HEALTH
Provide wholemeal cereals and dark green vegetables, which are quite high in iron. Offer orange juice with meals to increase iron absorption from nonmeat foods.

A VARIED DIET
Experiment with new foods. For packed lunches and after-school snacks, try hummus, which is made with chickpeas, and pâtés made of spinach and mushrooms.

COOKING METHODS
Prepare dishes like vegetable soups, stews and casseroles that can be frozen then reheated.

HOW THINGS TURNED OUT FOR LIZ AND SARAH

Liz was happy to see that Sarah's vegetarianism has made her more adventurous in her eating habits and even inspired her to try her hand at cooking for herself and her parents. Four nights a week, Liz still cooks a meat dish for herself and her husband and provides a vegetarian alternative for Sarah. But on these nights, she wishes that Sarah would refrain from criticising her parents' carnivorous tastes while at the table.

Cooking vegetables whole or in large pieces helps to preserve their nutritional content. There is less surface area exposed to the air and therefore less nutrients will be oxidised. Reserve the water after cooking vegetables and use it for making soups or gravies. Cooking vegetables in a wok (stir-frying) is a good way of preserving their nutrients because the vegetables are coated with a small amount of oil and are in contact with

METHODS OF COOKING

COOKING METHOD	BENEFITS	DISADVANTAGES
DEEP-FRYING		
Quick cooking in boiling fat.	Retains some vitamins.	Increases the fat content of foods.
DRY-FRYING		
Fat-free frying.	No fat added; good retention of vitamins and minerals.	Only suitable for foods containing some natural fat.
STIR-FRYING (WOK COOKING)		
Quick cooking method over high heat.	Crisp look and taste. Little fat is needed. Minimal vitamin loss.	High in salt if too much soya sauce is used.
MICROWAVING		
Cooking in a microwave oven (see box, p.150).	Minimal vitamin loss.	Uneven cooking with 'cold' and 'hot' spots in food.
BRAISING AND STEWING		
Slow cooking in liquid over several hours.	Improves flavour and texture of tough cuts of meat.	Vitamins leach into liquid but retention in stewing is better than in roasting.
GRILLING		
Quick cooking with dry heat.	No fat added; vitamins and minerals lost to pan sediments.	Charcoal or open-flame grilling of meats may induce the formation of carcinogens.
BOILING		
Cooking in large amounts of water.	Improves texture of tough vegetables.	Some vitamins lost to liquid.
POACHING		
Simmering in a little liquid.	No added fat.	Some vitamin loss.
STEAMING		
Cooking over steam that is converted from a little water.	Preserves most nutrients and flavour.	Need to watch cooking time carefully to prevent overcooking.
ROASTING		
Cooking with intense, dry heat.	Succulent meat; vegetables retain some vitamins.	Vitamin loss. Fat added to meat with the basting.
POT-ROASTING		
Slow baking in covered dish.	No added fat.	Loss of some vitamins.
PRESSURE COOKING		
Quick cooking at high temperature, minimal water.	Most vitamins and minerals preserved.	Timing difficult to control, which may cause overcooking.

heat for a minimum amount of time. Once cooked, vegetables should be served and eaten as soon as possible because they will begin to lose their nutritional content if allowed to stand.

MEAT

A rich source of protein, B vitamins, fats and minerals, meat can be a valuable part of a healthy diet. Protein does not diminish during cooking, and although vitamins and some minerals may leach into the cooking medium, you can use this to make soups, sauces and gravies.

Most meats, lamb and beef in particular, are high in saturated fat. Avoid excess fat by purchasing lean cuts of meat, such as fillet of beef. Make sure that you trim off all external fat. Meats that have been trimmed of fat require less cooking time than fatty meats. Therefore, reduce the normal cooking time by about 20 per cent. Rare meat will be more tender but always make sure that it is not undercooked (see box, below).

Use fat-free cooking methods, such as stewing, braising or grilling, as often as possible. When making a casserole, skim the fat off the top at regular intervals. Avoid frying meats, but, if you do, use olive or rapeseed oils, both of which are high in monounsaturated fats, instead of butter. Dry-fry fatty meats such as mince in non-stick pans, then pour away the fat that is released during cooking. Before roasting meat, place it on a rack inside the roasting tin. This allows the fat to drip from the meat during cooking.

POULTRY

Chicken is an excellent source of protein and contains relatively less fat than meat, especially when the skin is removed. Frozen chicken must be thoroughly defrosted. Before cooking, rinse the skin and the cavity and pat dry with kitchen paper. Always marinate pieces of chicken and meat in the refrigerator, not at room temperature.

Because of the risk of salmonella poisoning, poultry must never be undercooked. Place fatty birds like duck and goose on a rack in a roasting tin, then prick the skin before roasting. This allows some of the fat to escape. Chicken is extremely versatile and can be cooked in a variety of healthy ways, such as stir-frying, baking in foil or in baking parchment, or poaching (see p. 141).

FISH AND SHELLFISH

An especially healthy food, fish is high in protein and low in fat. Moreover, certain fish, such as salmon, trout, tuna, herrings, sardines and mackerel, are rich in omega-3

TESTING FOR DONENESS

Overcooked meat is dry and stringy. Eating undercooked meat and poultry, however, can be dangerous. Protein foods are particularly vulnerable to food-poisoning bacteria, which are killed if food is thoroughly cooked.

A reliable method of measuring the doneness of meat is to use a meat thermometer. It should be inserted into the thickest part of the flesh. Do not let it touch the bone, which conducts heat and will be hotter than the surrounding meat.

For rare beef and lamb, the meat thermometer will show 60°C (140°F); for medium-done it will show 70°C (160°F).

It is essential that pork be well cooked, because it may be contaminated with a parasite that causes the disease trichinosis. When pork is well-cooked, the thermometer will read 77°C (170°F).

Cooking poultry thoroughly will protect you against poisoning with salmonella bacteria. To check the doneness of a chicken, turkey, duck or goose, insert a poultry thermometer into the thickest part of the meat away from the bone. For a whole bird, the thermometer will read 82°C (180°F); for breast, thigh and wing pieces, it will read 77°C (170°F).

Another, more commonly used way of testing for doneness is to stick a skewer into the fleshiest part of the thigh and then let the juices run out. They should be clear, not pink. Alternatively, lift the whole bird with a two-pronged fork and check the juices as they run out of the cavity into the dish.

Fish is cooked when the eyes are opaque and the flesh flakes easily when tested with a fork.

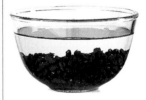

*DESTROYING TOXINS
Dried beans contain toxicants called lectins. If you eat improperly prepared beans, they can cause abdominal cramps, vomiting and death. Soaking the beans for at least 8 hours and boiling them for 10 minutes in fresh water before cooking destroys lectins.*

Dangerous microbes

If a food is contaminated with large numbers of bacteria, such as salmonella or listeria, it will cause food poisoning. But campylobacteria is dangerous in small numbers.

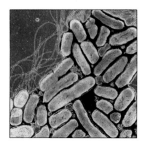

SALMONELLA BACTERIA
Infants, the elderly and people with weakened immune systems, such as cancer sufferers, are particularly vulnerable to salmonella poisoning.

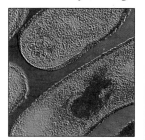

LISTERIA
Pregnant women should avoid soft cheeses and undercooked meat as this bacteria can be fatal for unborn babies.

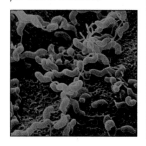

CAMPYLOBACTERIA
The bacteria live in animals and wild birds and are picked up by humans when touching animals or raw poultry.

fatty acids that may help to prevent heart disease. Shellfish are important sources of minerals, such as zinc.

All fresh fish should be scaled and gutted before cooking. Rinse fish under cold running water and pat dry with kitchen paper. Steaming, microwaving, grilling and poaching will retain the fish's moisture without adding much fat. Fish cooks perfectly in a microwave oven, but slash the skin to prevent pressure building up and splitting the fish. Baking fish in foil or baking parchment will help to retain flavour (see p. 141).

Scrub molluscs under cold running water and discard any that stay open when tapped lightly. Shellfish need to be boiled only for a few minutes. Throw away any clams, mussels or oysters that have not opened after cooking.

FOOD POISONING

Despite the advances in food processing and distribution that have helped to make food fresher and healthier, food poisoning is on the increase. In England and Wales, the increase of reported cases has been dramatic, rising from 14 253 in 1982 to 63 347 in 1992. In the United States, in 1978, there were 28 881 cases of food poisoning caused by the salmonella bacteria reported to the Centers for Disease Control and Prevention (CDC). By 1987, the number of reported cases had almost doubled. The CDC estimates the number of people that are actually affected by food poisoning to be even higher.

Careless handling of food before and after cooking and insufficient heating will cause bacteria to grow at an alarming rate. But food poisoning can be prevented with careful preparation, storage and cooking.

Causes of food poisoning

Bacteria are single-cell organisms that are invisible to the naked eye. Given suitable temperatures and conditions, bacteria can double their numbers in 20 minutes. Bacteria are transferred to humans either from food – poultry and eggs are typical examples of salmonella carriers – or from the excrement of infected people or animals.

The most common disease-producing bacteria belong to the salmonella and camphylobacter groups. These bacteria can multiply with tremendous rapidity in the intestines and cause widespread inflammation. Some types of bacteria – for example,

CONTROLLING BACTERIA

Meat, poultry and eggs all harbour bacteria that can be destroyed when heated properly. If a food is kept at a temperature within the 'danger zone', however, it may cause serious illness when eaten.

▶ *Cooking temperatures (74°C/165°F to 100°C/ 212°F) destroy most bacteria. The higher the temperature, the less time needed to kill bacteria.*

▶ *Warming temperatures (60°C/140°F to 74°C/165°F) prevent the growth of bacteria, but they still survive.*

▶ *Bacteria grow rapidly and produce toxins in temperatures between 16°C/61°F and 49°C/120°F.*

▶ *Cold temperatures (0°C/32°F to 6°C/43°F) allow the slow growth of bacteria.*

▶ *Freezing temperatures (-18°C/0°F to -10°C to 14°F) prevent the growth of bacteria but do not kill them.*

Staphylococcus aureus and *Clostridium botulinum* – produce toxins that cause food poisoning upon swallowing.

Symptoms

Nausea, diarrhoea, vomiting and stomach pain are common symptoms of food poisoning. Severe cases may also include shock and collapse. Botulism toxin, however, has a different set of symptoms that affect the central nervous system and cause problems with speech, visual disturbances, muscle paralysis and vomiting.

Viruses do not multiply in foods but they do contaminate certain foods from seabeds polluted by untreated sewage. There can be serious consequences from eating raw shellfish and raw fish (sushi). Always buy fish from a reputable supplier.

What to do for food poisoning

With the exception of poisoning from mushrooms, from *Escherichia Coli* (type 0157:H7), or botulism poisoning, episodes of food poisoning, although unpleasant, are rarely fatal. Someone who is suffering from food poisoning should avoid solid foods until the symptoms clear up and drink plenty of fluids to rehydrate the body. Babies, toddlers and elderly people are particularly at risk from dehydration. An oral rehydration solution, which contains a mixture of salt and sugar, is the best way to treat dehydration. You can buy one from a chemist or make your own – one teaspoon of salt and eight teaspoons of sugar in 1 litre (1¾ pints) of water. Lethargy and weakness are common until the poisoning clears the body, so rest will be necessary.

For severe vomiting and diarrhoea, or if the affected person collapses, seek medical help immediately. The sufferer may be required to provide a faecal sample so that it can be analysed to identify the cause. If you have kept a sample of the food responsible, it should also be sent away for analysis. If a restaurant is responsible, inform your local environmental health department.

FOOD POISONING SYMPTOMS

Reactions to food poisoning can vary, but they are mostly dependent on the extent of the contamination to which the food has been exposed. The most common causes of food poisoning are shown in the chart below.

SYMPTOMS	ONSET	AFFECTED FOODS
ESCHERICHIA COLI (TYPE 0157:H7) ✳✳✳		
Abdominal cramps, diarrhoea, vomiting, low-grade fever.	12 to 72 hours.	Undercooked hamburger or roast beef, unpasteurised milk.
CHEMICAL POISONING ✳✳✳		
Diarrhoea, vomiting.	Within 30 minutes.	Seafood from polluted water.
STAPHYLOCOCCI ✳✳		
Vomiting, nausea, diarrhoea, abdominal cramps.	Few minutes to 6 hours.	Meat, poultry, egg and dairy dishes.
CLOSTRIDIUM PERFRINGENS ✳✳		
Diarrhoea, abdominal cramps.	6 to 12 hours.	Meat, gravies, stuffing.
CLOSTRIDIUM BOTULINUM (BOTULISM) ✳✳✳		
Slurred speech, blurred vision, paralysis. Death can occur from respiratory failure.	18 to 36 hours.	Improperly canned foods, foods contaminated by flies.
SALMONELLA ORGANISMS ✳		
Diarrhoea, vomiting, fever, abdominal cramps, headache.	8 to 36 hours.	Poultry, eggs, raw meat, dairy products, shellfish.
VIRUSES (HEPATITIS A) ✳✳		
Diarrhoea, vomiting, fever, jaundice. Severe cases can be fatal.	12 to 48 hours.	Contaminated seafood, especially raw shellfish.
SHIGELLA ORGANISMS ✳		
Abdominal cramps, fever, diarrhoea.	2 to 3 days.	Dairy products, tuna, poultry, potato salad.
CAMPYLOBACTERIA ✳		
Abdominal cramps, fever, diarrhoea, sometimes bloody stools.	2 to 6 days.	Meat, poultry, milk.
LISTERIA MONOCYTOGENES ✳✳		
Headache, nausea, fever.	4 to 6 hours to several days.	Soft cheese, seafood, pâté.

✳ Rest and take plenty of fluids   ✳✳ See your doctor if symptoms persist   ✳✳✳ Seek medical help immediately

Natural toxins

A wide variety of foods contain natural poisons that are harmful only if eaten in large amounts. Small fish and shellfish feeding off algae may also ingest algal toxins. These accumulate in their flesh and in the flesh of larger predatory fish such as snapper and sea bass. The toxins can reach levels that are poisonous to humans. Ciguatera poisoning, which is caused by ingesting fish that are contaminated with algal toxins, occurs occasionally in the United States; the symptoms include cramps and numb and tingling lips. Poisoning by algal toxins is extremely rare in the United Kingdom. Shellfish are regularly monitored for toxins in both the United Kingdom and the United States.

The potato also harbours a natural toxin, solanine, which is usually present in low levels. High levels of this toxin are found in the green parts of potatoes, in sprouted potatoes and in potatoes exposed to light. Because this toxin is not destroyed by cooking, the green parts must be discarded.

CONVERSION TABLES

The tables below provide rounded-up equivalents in weight. Following one or the other of the charts when preparing a recipe will provide a successful result. However, it is important to stick to either metric or imperial measurements, and not to switch from one to the other within a recipe or the proportions will change slightly.

Measuring cups in ¼, ⅓, ½ and 1 cup sizes are used for dry ingredients

Teaspoons and tablespoons can be used for both liquid and dry ingredients

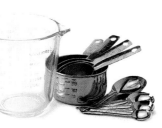

A 600 ml (1 pint) measuring jug is useful when measuring large amounts. Make sure you check the volume of liquid at eye level

MEASURING CUPS

In the United States, many dry ingredients are measured by volume rather than weight. The standard US cup holds 225 millilitres (8 fluid ounces) of liquid. As a guide for any UK cooks using an American cookery book, a selection of frequently used foods are shown below with their equivalent metric and imperial weights per US cup.

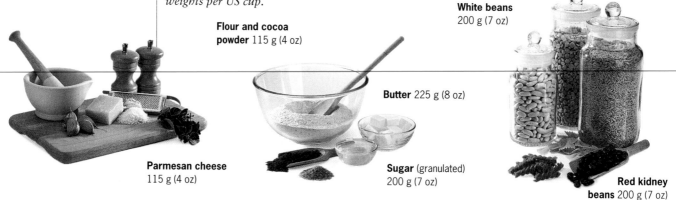

Flour and cocoa powder 115 g (4 oz)

White beans 200 g (7 oz)

Rice 200 g (7 oz)

Butter 225 g (8 oz)

Parmesan cheese 115 g (4 oz)

Sugar (granulated) 200 g (7 oz)

Red kidney beans 200 g (7 oz)

WEIGHT CHART

DRY MEASURES		LIQUID MEASURES	
METRIC	IMPERIAL	METRIC	IMPERIAL
15 g	½ oz	5 ml	1 teaspoon
25 g	1 oz	15 ml	1 tablespoon
40 g	1½ oz	30 ml	2 tbsp
55 g	2 oz	60 ml	4 tbsp
70 g	2½ oz	100 ml	3½ fl oz
85 g	3 oz	125 ml	4 fl oz
100 g	3½ oz	150 ml	5 fl oz (¼ pint)
115 g	4 oz	175 ml	6 fl oz
140 g	5 oz	200 ml	7 fl oz
175 g	6 oz	225 ml	8 fl oz
200 g	7 oz	300 ml	10 fl oz (½ pint)
225 g	8 oz	350 ml	12 fl oz
280 g	10 oz	425 ml	15 fl oz (¾ pint)
350 g	12 oz	450 ml	16 fl oz
450 g	16 oz (1 lb)	600 ml	20 fl oz (1 pint)

TEMPERATURES

°C	°F	GAS MARK
80	150	Keep warm
90	175	Keep warm
100	200	Keep warm
110	225	¼
120	250	½ cool
140	275	1
150	300	2
160	325	3 moderate
180	350	4
190	375	5
200	400	6 hot
220	425	7
230	450	8
240	475	9
250	500	10 very hot

INDEX

ACKNOWLEDGMENTS

Carroll & Brown Limited
would like to thank
Dr Frazer Anderson,
   Musculoskeletal Unit,
   Freeman Hospital,
   Newcastle upon Tyne

Mike Rayner,
Oxford University,
   Department of Public Health
     & Primary Care,
   Radcliffe Infirmary,
   Oxford

James Arnold
Ellen Dupont
Sue Mimms

British Heart Foundation
Child Growth Foundation
The Coeliac Society
Ealing Active Leisure,
   London Borough of Ealing
The Shellfish Association
The Vegetarian Society
Zenith International Ltd

Writers
Anita Bean, Susan Broadman,
Helen Crawley, Moya De Wet,
Samar El-Daher, Jeanette Ewin,
Miranda Holden, Judy Marshel,
William Murray, Roger Newman-
Turner, Mark Ravenhill,
Judy Sadgrove, Stephen Ulph

Photograph sources
8 Popperfoto
9 Popperfoto
10 Range Pictures
11 Zefa
12 Niall McInerney
33 Matt Meadows/Peter Arnold
   Inc/SPL
44 David Parker/SPL
54 National Library of Medicine/SPL
66 (Top left) Image Bank/David de
   Lossy, (Bottom left) Eric Grave/
   SPL, (Bottom right) National
   Medical Slide Bank
69 (Left and right) Professor P. Motta,
   Department of Anatomy,
   University 'La Sapienza',
   Rome/SPL
80 Pictures Colour Library
91 (Top) Image Bank/Gerald
   Brimacombe, (Bottom) Mike
   Newton/The Robert Harding
   Picture Library
102 CNRI/SPL
110 CNRI/SPL
114 Pictures Colour Library
124 Peter Tizzard
135 (Top) Giraudon/Bridgeman Art
   Library, (Bottom) Niall
   McInerney
154 (Top) A.B. Dowsett/SPL, (Centre)
   Institut Pasteur/CNR/SPL,
   (Bottom) Moredun Animal Health
   Ltd/SPL

Illustrators
Joanna Cameron
Jane Craddock-Watson
Eugene Fleury
John Geary
Christine Pilsworth
Paul Williams
Angela Wood

Charts
Clive Bruton
Lee Maunder
Nick Roland

Photographic assistants
Nick Allen
Ian Boddy
Alex Hansen
Sid Sideris

Picture researcher
Sandra Schneider

Food preparation
Maddalena Bastianelli
Eric Treuille

Research
Laura Price

Index
Madeline Weston

Note
Metric and imperial measures are given
throughout except when calculating measures
of nutrients, which are given in metric only.

75-001-05